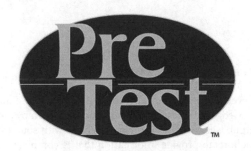

Psychiatry

PreTest™ Self-Assessment and Review

Notice

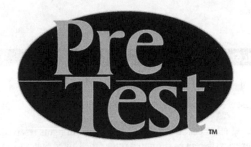

Psychiatry

PreTest™ Self-Assessment and Review

13th Edition

Debra L. Klamen, MD, MHPE, FAPA
Associate Dean, Education and Curriculum
Professor and Chair, Department of Medical Education
Southern Illinois University
Springfield, Illinois

Philip Pan, MD
Director, Outpatient Services
Assistant Professor, Department of Psychiatry
Southern Illinois University
Springfield, Illinois

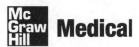

New York   Chicago   San Francisco   Lisbon   London   Madrid   Mexico City
Milan   New Delhi   San Juan   Seoul   Singapore   Sydney   Toronto

The **McGraw-Hill** Companies

Psychiatry: PreTest™ Self-Assessment and Review, 13th Edition

2 3 4 5 6 7 8 9 0   DOC/DOC   17 16 15 14 13

ISBN 978-0-07-176101-7
MHID 0-07-176101-2

This book was set in Berkeley by Cenveo Publisher Services.
The editors were Kirsten Funk and Cindy Yoo.
The production supervisor was Sherri Souffrance.
Project management was provided by Ridhi Mathur, Cenveo Publisher Services.
RR Donnelley was printer and binder.

This book is printed on acid-free paper.

Library of Congress Cataloging-in-Publication Data

Klamen, Debra L.
    Psychiatry : PreTest self-assessment & review.—13th ed. / Debra
L. Klamen, Philip Pan.
        p. ; cm.
    Includes bibliographical references and index.
    ISBN-13: 978-0-07-176101-7 (pbk. : alk. paper)
    ISBN-10: 0-07-176101-2 (pbk. : alk. paper)
    I. Pan, Philip.   II. Title.
    [DNLM: 1. Mental Disorders—Examination Questions.
    2. Psychotherapy—Examination Questions. WM 18.2]
    616.890076—dc23

                                            2011035293

McGraw-Hill books are available at special quantity discounts to use as premiums and sales promotions, or for use in corporate training programs. To contact a representative please e-mail us at bulksales@mcgraw-hill.com.

Student Reviewers

Amanda Cooper
Fourth Year Medical Student
New York College of Osteopathic Medicine
Class of 2012

Robin Hanson
Fourth Year Medical Student
UMDNJ School of Osteopathic Medicine
Class of 2011

Akinbowale Oyalowo
Fourth Year Medical Student
University of Maryland
Class of 2012

Tony Tao
Fourth Year Medical Student
SUNY Downstate Medical Center
Class of 2010

Xiaolin (Lynn) Zhang
Fourth Year Medical Student
UMDNJ Robert Wood Johnson Medical School
Class of 2010

Contents

Mood Disorders

Anxiety, Somatoform, and Dissociative Disorders

Personality Disorders, Human Sexuality, and Miscellaneous Syndromes

Substance-Related Disorders

Psychopharmacology and Other Somatic Therapies

Law and Ethics in Psychiatry

Introduction

Psychiatry: PreTest™ Self-Assessment and Review, 13th edition, has been designed to provide medical students and international medical graduates with a comprehensive and convenient instrument for self-assessment and review. The 500 questions provided have been written to parallel the topics, format, and degree of difficulty of the questions contained in the United States Medical Licensing Examination (USMLE) Step 2CK.

Each question in the book is accompanied by an answer, a paragraph explanation, and a specific page reference to a standard textbook or other major resource. These books have been carefully selected for their educational excellence and ready availability in most libraries. A bibliography listing all the sources used in the book follows the last chapter. Diagnostic nomenclature is that of the fourth edition of the *Diagnostic and Statistical Manual of Mental Disorders (DSM-IV-TR).*

One effective way to use this book is to allow yourself one minute to answer each question in a given chapter and to mark your answer beside the question. By following this suggestion, you will be training yourself for the time limits commonly imposed by examinations. For multiple-choice questions, the **one best** response to each question should be selected. For matching sets, a group of questions will be preceded by a list of lettered options. For each question in the matching set, select **one** lettered option that is **most** closely associated with the question.

Since there are few absolutes in clinical practice, remember to simply choose the best possible answer. There are no "trick" questions intended. Rather, each question has been designed to address a significant topic. Some important topics are deliberately duplicated in other sections of the book when this is deemed helpful. All questions apply to the treatment of adults unless otherwise indicated.

When you have finished answering the questions in a chapter, you should spend as much time as you need to verify your answers and to absorb the explanations. Although you should pay special attention to the explanations for the questions you answered incorrectly, you should read every explanation. Each explanation is written to reinforce and supplement the information tested by the question. When you identify a gap in your fund of knowledge, or if you simply need more information about a topic, you should consult and study the references indicated.

Evaluation, Assessment, and Diagnosis

Questions

1. A 32-year-old woman is seen in an outpatient psychiatric clinic for the chief complaint of a depressed mood for 4 months. During the interview, she gives very long, complicated explanations and many unnecessary details before finally answering the original questions. Which of the following psychiatric findings best describes this style of train of thought?

a. Loose association
b. Circumstantiality
c. Neologism
d. Perseveration
e. Flight of ideas

2. A 23-year-old man comes to the psychiatrist with a chief complaint of a depressed mood. He is very anxious and obviously uncomfortable in the physician's office. Which of the following actions should be used to help develop rapport with this patient?

a. Inform the patient that his problem is simple and easily fixed.
b. Express compassion with the difficult position the patient is in.
c. Tell the patient that you too are nervous when you see new patients.
d. Ask the patient why he is so unusually anxious about seeing a psychiatrist.
e. Get right to the patient's complaint so that the patient can leave as soon as possible.

3. An 18-year-old man is seen by a psychiatrist in the emergency room. During the history, the patient is asked to describe his mood. He answers the following, "My mood is flextitating, I am up and down." He notes that he believes that the CIA has been listening to his thoughts through the walls of his home. Which of the following findings would be listed on a report of this patient's mental status examination?

a. Clang association, delusions of grandeur
b. Thought blocking, auditory hallucination
c. No apparent thought disorder
d. Tangentiality, labile affect
e. Neologism, paranoid delusion

4. A 56-year-old man has been hospitalized for a myocardial infarction. Two days after admission, he awakens in the middle of the night and screams that there is a man standing by the window in his room. When the nurse enters the room and turns on a light, the patient is relieved to learn that the "man" was actually a drape by the window. This misperception of reality is best described by which of the following psychiatric terms?

a. Delusion
b. Hallucination
c. Illusion
d. Projection
e. Dementia

5. A 22-year-old woman is seen by a psychiatrist in the emergency room after she is found walking in the middle of a busy street with no shoes on. During her interview she is asked to count backwards from 100 by 7s. Which of the following best describes the cognitive functions being tested by this request?

a. Orientation
b. Immediate memory
c. Fund of knowledge
d. Concentration
e. Abstract reasoning

6. A 28-year-old woman is admitted to the hospital secondary to a bacterial pneumonia. Her white blood cell count is extremely low because she has been receiving chemotherapy for lymphoma. The second night in the hospital, she begins crying inconsolably, though she is unable to tell the nurse why. Forty minutes later, she pulls out her IV and begins screaming that people are trying to hurt her. Several hours later she is found to be difficult to arouse and is disoriented. Which of the following is the most likely diagnosis?

a. Major depression
b. Brief reactive psychosis
c. Acute manic episode
d. Delirium
e. Acute stress disorder

7. A 52-year-old man is sent to see a psychiatrist after he is disciplined at his job because he consistently turns in his assignments late. He insists that he is not about to turn in anything until it is "perfect, unlike all of my colleagues." He has few friends because he annoys them with his demands for "precise timeliness" and because of his lack of emotional warmth. This has been a lifelong pattern for the patient, though he refuses to believe the problems have anything to do with his personal behavior. Which of the following is the most likely diagnosis for this patient?

a. Obsessive-compulsive disorder
b. Obsessive-compulsive personality disorder
c. Borderline personality disorder
d. Bipolar disorder, mixed state
e. Anxiety disorder not otherwise specified

8. A 23-year-old woman comes to the psychiatrist because she "cannot get out of the shower." She tells the psychiatrist that she has been unable to go to her job as a secretary for the past 3 weeks because it takes her at least 4 hours to shower. She describes an elaborate ritual in which she must make sure that each part of her body has been scrubbed three times, in exactly the same order each time. She notes that her hands are raw and bloody from all the scrubbing. She states that she hates what she is doing to herself but becomes unbearably anxious each time she tries to stop. She notes that she has always taken long showers, but the problem has been worsening steadily for the past 5 months. She denies problems with friends or at work, other than the problems that currently are keeping her from going to work. Which of the following is the most likely diagnosis?

a. Attention-deficit hyperactivity disorder
b. Obsessive-compulsive disorder
c. Obsessive-compulsive personality disorder
d. Separation anxiety disorder
e. Brief psychotic disorder

9. A 37-year-old man with chronic schizophrenia is brought to see a new psychiatrist for treatment. While taking the history, the psychiatrist finds that the patient functions with a flat affect and circumstantial speech all the time. He has few friends. He is able to hold a menial job at the halfway house where he lives, and his behavior is not influenced by delusions or hallucinations currently. What should the psychiatrist rate the patient on Axis V (global assessment of functioning)?

a. >95
b. 70
c. 55
d. 30
e. 15

Questions 10 to 13

Match each of the following vignettes with the most likely diagnosis. Each lettered option may be used once, more than once, or not at all.

a. Panic disorder
b. Generalized anxiety disorder
c. Schizoid personality disorder
d. Schizotypal personality disorder
e. Anxiety secondary to a general medical condition
f. Factitious disorder
g. Malingering
h. Schizophreniform disorder
i. Schizophrenia

10. A 28-year-old man comes to the psychiatrist because his employer required it. The patient says that he does not know why the employer required it—that his job is good and that he likes it because it requires him to sit in front of a computer screen all day. He notes he has one friend whom he has had for more than 20 years and "doesn't need anyone else." The friend lives in another state and the patient has not seen him for at least a year. The patient denies any psychotic symptoms. His eye contact is poor and his affect is almost flat.

11. A 42-year-old woman is admitted to the hospital for complaints of abdominal pain. Her history notes that her mother was a nurse and she herself is trained as a phlebotomist. On physical examination, she presents with multiple abdominal scars and marked abdominal tenderness. The patient is evasive when asked where she had the surgeries, but she can describe in great detail what was done in each.

12. An 18-year-old man is brought to the emergency room by his college roommate, after the roommate discovered that the patient had not left his room for the past 3 days, neither to eat nor to go to the bathroom. The roommate noted that the patient was kind of "weird." Mental status examination reveals that the patient has auditory hallucinations of two voices commenting upon his behavior. The patient's parents note that their son has always been somewhat of a loner and unpopular, but otherwise did fairly well in school.

13. A 32-year-old woman comes to the psychiatrist with a chief complaint of anxiety. She notes that she worries about paying the mortgage on time, whether or not she will get stuck in traffic and be late for appointments, her husband's and daughter's health, and the war in Iraq. She notes that she has always been anxious, but since the birth of her daughter 2 years ago, the anxiety has worsened to the point that she feels she cannot function as well as she did previously.

14. A 23-year-old woman comes to the emergency room with the chief complaint that she has been hearing voices for 7 months. Besides the hallucinations, she has the idea that the radio is giving her special messages. When asked the meaning of the proverb "People in glass houses should not throw stones," the patient replies, "Because the windows would break." Which of the following mental status findings does this patient display?

a. Poverty of content
b. Concrete thinking
c. Flight of ideas
d. Loose associations
e. Delirium

15. A 22-year-old woman is seen in the emergency room after a suicide attempt. She swallowed 10 aspirin tablets in the presence of her mother, with whom she had just had an argument. The patient has a long history of cutting herself superficially with razor blades, which her psychiatrist of the last 5 years confirms by telephone. The patient currently lives in a stable environment (a halfway house) where she has been for 3 years. Which of the following options is the best course of action for the physician in the emergency room assuming that the patient has been medically cleared?

a. Admit the patient involuntarily.
b. Admit the patient voluntarily.
c. Keep the patient in an observation room for 24 hours in the emergency room.
d. Discharge the patient to outpatient therapy after meeting with the patient's mother.
e. Discharge the patient back to outpatient therapy and the halfway house.

16. A 69-year-old man is brought to see his physician by his wife. She notes that over the past year he has experienced a slow, stepwise decline in his cognitive functioning. One year ago she felt his thinking was "as good as it always had been," but now he gets lost around the house and can't remember simple directions. The patient insists that he feels fine, though he is depressed about his loss of memory. He is eating and sleeping well. Which of the following is the most likely diagnosis?

a. Multi-infarct dementia
b. Mood disorder secondary to a general medical condition
c. Schizoaffective disorder
d. Delirium
e. Major depression

17. A 24-year-old woman comes to a psychiatrist with the chief complaint of hearing voices. During the interview, the patient is intermittently tearful when she speaks of hearing the voices. She states that she has been feeling sad for the past 6 weeks, and she appears this way to the interviewer as well. During the entire interview the patient never appears other than sad. How would this patient's mood and affect be characterized in a mental status examination?

a. Mood—constricted   Affect—flat, incongruent
b. Mood—euthymic   Affect—full range, congruent
c. Mood—dysphoric   Affect—constricted, congruent
d. Mood—dysphoric   Affect—labile, congruent
e. Mood—flat   Affect—dysphoric

18. A 6-year-old girl is brought to the physician by her mother, who says the child has been falling behind at school. She notes that the girl did not speak until the age of 4, though her hearing was tested at age 3 and found to be normal. She is friendly at school, but is unable to complete most tasks, even when aided. She is noted to have a very short attention span and occasional temper tantrums at school and at home. She enjoys playing with her toys at home. Which of the following tests would be most helpful in establishing the diagnosis?

a. Electroencephalogram (EEG)
b. Beck depression test
c. IQ testing
d. Complete blood count (CBC)
e. Lumbar puncture

Questions 19 to 21

19. A 30-year-old man is brought to the emergency room after threatening to kill his 19-year-old girlfriend after she told him she was breaking up with him. The patient smells strongly of alcohol. The patient is from a high socioeconomic status and reports many social supports. Which of the following pairs of factors make this patient's risk of violent behavior higher?

a. His age and his alcohol use
b. His alcohol use and the impending breakup with the girlfriend
c. The impending breakup with the girlfriend and his high socioeconomic status
d. His high socioeconomic status and the presence of many social supports in his life
e. The age difference of the couple and a verbal threat of violence by the patient

20. The patient above becomes physically violent in the emergency room, attempting to strike a nurse and struggling with security. Which of the following actions should the psychiatrist take now?

a. Order full leather restraints.
b. Admit the patient to the inpatient psychiatry unit.
c. Offer the patient 5 mg of haloperidol PO.
d. Attempt to find out why the patient is so upset.
e. Assist security in restraining the patient.

21. The patient in question 19 is eventually placed in full leather restraints. He struggles against them and screams racial slurs repeatedly. What would be the next most appropriate action for the psychiatrist to take?

a. Give haloperidol 5 mg IM and lorazepam 2 mg IM.
b. Start an IV and give diazepam 5 mg IVP.
c. Draw a blood toxicology screen to look for other drugs of abuse.
d. Give a loading dose of carbamazepine.
e. Send the patient for an MRI of his head.

22. A psychiatrist is seeing a patient in his outpatient practice. The patient treats the psychiatrist as if he were unreliable and punitive, though he had not been either. The patient's father was an alcoholic who often did not show up to pick her up from school and frequently hit her. The psychiatrist begins to feel as if he must overprotect the patient and treat her gingerly. Which of the following psychological mechanisms best describes the psychiatrist's behavior?

a. Reaction formation
b. Projection
c. Countertransference
d. Identification with the aggressor
e. Illusion

23. A 65-year-old man, who had been hospitalized for an acute pneumonia 3 days previously, begins screaming for his nurse, stating that "there are people in the room out to get me." He then gets out of bed and begins pulling out his IV line. On examination, he alternates between agitation and somnolence. He is not oriented to time or place. His vital signs are as follows: pulse, 126 beats/minute; respiration, 32 breaths/minute; blood pressure (BP), 80/58 mm/Hg; temperature, 39.2°C (102.5°F). Which of the following diagnoses best fits this patient's clinical picture?

a. Dementia
b. Schizophreniform disorder
c. Fugue state
d. Delirium
e. Brief psychotic episode

24. A 23-year-old man presents to the emergency room with the history of a fever up to 38°C (100.5°F) intermittently over the past 2 weeks, a persistent cough, and a 10-lb weight loss in the past month. He notes that he has also been growing increasingly forgetful for the past month and that his thinking is "not always clear." He has gotten lost twice recently while driving. Which of the following diagnostic tests will be most helpful with this patient?

a. EEG
b. Liver function tests
c. Thyroid function tests
d. HIV antibody test
e. Skull X-ray

25. A 19-year-old woman presents to the emergency room with the chief complaint of a depressed mood for 2 weeks. She notes that since her therapist went on vacation she has experienced suicidal ideation, crying spells, and an increased appetite. She states that she has left 40 messages on the therapist's answering machine telling him that she is going to kill herself and that it would serve him right for leaving her. Physical examination reveals multiple well-healed scars and cigarette burns on the anterior aspect of both forearms. Which of the following diagnoses best fits this patient's clinical presentation?

a. Dysthymic disorder
b. Bipolar disorder
c. Panic disorder
d. Borderline personality disorder
e. Schizoaffective disorder

26. A 29-year-old man is brought to the emergency room by his wife after he woke up with paralysis of his right arm. The patient reports that the day before, he had gotten into a verbal altercation with his mother over her intrusiveness in his life. The patient notes that he has always had mixed feelings about his mother, but that people should always respect their mothers above all else. Which of the following diagnoses best fits this patient's clinical picture?

a. Major depression
b. Conversion disorder
c. Histrionic personality disorder
d. Fugue state
e. Adjustment disorder

27. A 28-year-old business executive sees her physician because she is having difficulty in her new position, as it requires her to do frequent public speaking. She states that she is terrified she will do or say something that will cause her extreme embarrassment. The patient says that when she must speak in public, she becomes extremely anxious and her heart beats uncontrollably. Based on this clinical picture, which of the following is the most likely diagnosis?

a. Panic disorder
b. Avoidant personality disorder
c. Specific phobia
d. Agoraphobia
e. Social phobia

28. A diagnostic test has a sensitivity of 64% and a specificity of 99%. Such a test would carry the risk of which kind of problem?

a. High relative risk
b. Low likelihood ratio
c. False negatives
d. False positives
e. Low power

29. A 56-year-old man is brought to the physician's office by his wife because she has noted a personality change during the past 3 months. While the patient is being interviewed, he answers every question with the same three words. Which of the following symptoms best fits this patient's behavior?

a. Negative symptoms
b. Disorientation
c. Concrete thinking
d. Perseveration
e. Circumstantiality

30. A 32-year-old patient is being interviewed in his physician's office. He eventually answers each question, but he gives long answers with a great deal of tedious and unnecessary detail before doing so. Which of the following symptoms best describes this patient's presentation?

a. Blocking
b. Tangentiality
c. Circumstantiality
d. Looseness of associations
e. Flight of ideas

31. An 18-year-old man is brought to the emergency room by the police after he is found walking along the edge of a high building. In the emergency room, he mumbles to himself and appears to be responding to internal stimuli. When asked open-ended questions, he suddenly stops his answer in the middle of a sentence, as if he has forgotten what to say. Which of the following symptoms best describes this last behavior?

a. Incongruent affect
b. Blocking
c. Perseveration
d. Tangentiality
e. Thought insertion

32. A 26-year-old woman with panic disorder notes that during the middle of one of her attacks she feels as if she is disconnected from the world, as though it were artificial or distant. Which of the following terms best describes this symptom?

a. Mental status change
b. Illusion
c. Retardation of thought
d. Depersonalization
e. Derealization

33. A patient with a chronic psychotic disorder is convinced that she has caused a recent earthquake because she was bored and wishing for something exciting to occur. Which of the following symptoms most closely describes this patient's thoughts?

a. Thought broadcasting
b. Magical thinking
c. Echolalia
d. Nihilism
e. Obsession

Questions 34 to 37

Match the following diagnosis with the description that best fits it. Each lettered option may be used once, more than once, or not at all.

a. Conscious, intentional production of symptoms with primary gain
b. Conscious, intentional production of symptoms with secondary gain
c. Unconscious, unintentional production of symptoms
d. Conscious, unintentional production of symptoms
e. Unconscious intentional production of symptoms

34. Malingering

35. Factitious disorder

36. Somatization disorder

37. Conversion disorder

38. A 45-year-old man with a chronic psychotic disorder is interviewed after being admitted to a psychiatric unit. He mimics the examiner's body posture and movements during the interview. Which of the following terms best characterizes this patient's symptom?

a. Folie à deux
b. Dereistic thinking
c. Echolalia
d. Echopraxia
e. Fugue

Questions 39 to 41

Match the patient's symptoms with the most appropriate diagnostic axis. Each lettered option may be used once, more than once, or not at all.

a. Axis I
b. Axis II
c. Axis III
d. Axis IV
e. Axis V

39. A 32-year-old man complains of depressed mood, poor concentration, a 25-lb weight gain, and hypersomnia. He is subsequently diagnosed with hypothyroidism.

40. A 46-year-old college professor has been unable to go to work for the past 6 weeks because of his psychiatric symptoms.

41. A 23-year-old woman works in a sheltered workshop. She is unable to make change for a dollar or read beyond a second-grade level. She has a genetic makeup of 47 chromosomes with three copies of chromosome 21.

Questions 42 to 45

Match the following vignettes with the diagnoses they best describe. Each lettered option may be used once, more than once, or not at all.

a. Oppositional defiant disorder
b. Conduct disorder
c. Antisocial personality disorder
d. Malingering

42. A 13-year-old boy is expelled from school because he has been bullying several classmates. He has been suspended previously for setting a fire at the school in a classroom garbage can. His parents note that he lies without seeming to feel any guilt. He has been running away from home frequently, and truancy from school has been a chronic concern since he was 10.

43. A 22-year-old man is arrested after he was caught forging a neighbor's check which he stole from her purse. He was kicked out of his parents' house several years previously because he repeatedly stole from them, lied about his whereabouts, and abused drugs in their presence. He seems completely unconcerned about all this behavior.

44. A 24-year-old woman comes to the emergency department complaining of "the worst belly pain I have ever felt." Although physical examination is normal, the woman continues to insist that she is in terrible pain and that she needs strong pain medication to tolerate it. It is later discovered she has visited three emergency departments in the city in the past week with the same complaint and demand for narcotics.

45. A 12-year-old girl is brought to the psychiatrist by her parents, who state that they are at their wits' end because of her behavior. They note that for at least the past year, she has been extremely temperamental. She deliberately goes out of her way to annoy people and is very easily annoyed by others. When she becomes angry, she rapidly becomes spiteful and vindictive. The girl denies any of this and blames her parents for their poor parenting skills as responsible for any problems she may be having.

Questions 46 to 52

Match the following vignettes with the diagnoses they best describe. Each lettered option may be used once, more than once, or not at all.

a. Anticholinergic syndrome
b. Neuroleptic malignant syndrome
c. Acute dystonic reaction
d. Akathisia
e. Serotonin syndrome
f. Thyrotoxicosis
g. Malignant hyperthermia

46. A 26-year-old woman presents with ventricular tachycardia, metabolic acidosis, respiratory acidosis, muscle rigidity, and a temperature of 102°F. Her family notes that this kind of reaction to the medication runs in her family.

47. A 22-year-old man presents with extreme rigidity, altered mental status, temperature of 104°F, and a highly elevated CPK.

48. A 45-year-old man presents to the emergency room with a temperature of 105°F, tachycardia, arrhythmia, vomiting, diarrhea, and dehydration. He was noted to have been recently ill with pneumonia but was thought to be recovering.

49. A 65-year-old woman is brought to the emergency room by her husband. She is delirious, and her husband notes that before she became that way she complained of blurry vision, dry mouth, and constipation.

50. A 37-year-old man presents with headache, confusion, shivering, sweating, hypertension, nausea, diarrhea, and hyperreflexia.

51. A 29-year-old woman presents to the emergency room because she is unable to move her head, which remains tilted off to one side. (A lateral flexion contracture of the cervical spine musculature.)

52. A 32-year-old woman presents with restlessness and motor agitation. When questioned, she notes that "I feel like I have to move." She denies auditory or visual hallucinations.

Questions 53 to 62

Match the following characteristic findings on EEG with the clinical vignette that mostly likely will produce them. Each lettered option may be used once, more than once, or not at all.

a. Diffuse slowing of background rhythms
b. Increase in amplitude or voltage of theta activity
c. Generalized paroxysmal activity and spike discharges
d. Epileptiform discharge
e. Periodic lateralizing epileptiform discharges
f. Decreased alpha activity; increased voltage of theta and delta waves
g. Increased alpha activity in frontal area of brain; overall slow alpha activity
h. Marked decrease in alpha activity
i. Triphasic waves (generalized synchronous waves occurring in brief runs)
j. Generalized periodic sharp waves

53. A 21-year-old man suddenly loses consciousness and falls to the floor. He is witnessed to have a series of tonic-clonic contractions of his arms and legs. A short time afterwards, he awakens, but is drowsy and confused.

54. A 46-year-old man is brought to the emergency room after his friends note that he is having difficulties with coordination and writing. On examination he is disoriented and exhibits asterixis as well as jaundice.

55. A 72-year-old woman is found at home by her daughter and brought to the hospital. The daughter notes her mother seems confused, is much more irritable than her usual personality, is having trouble concentrating, and is lethargic. Laboratory examinations show a severe electrolyte imbalance.

56. A 52-year-old woman is brought to the emergency room after she collapsed at work. She has a long history of hypertension which has not been well controlled. In the emergency room she is noted to have a complete loss of muscle control in both her right arm and leg.

57. A 41-year-old man is diagnosed with a rapidly fatal disease. He dies within 6 months of the diagnosis. His disease started with some behavioral and personality changes, followed by a rapidly progressive dementia and episodes of myoclonus.

58. A 32-year-old man injects an illicit substance into his vein. He immediately has a sharp decrease in respiration, as well as pinpoint pupils. It requires more and more of the substance to allow the man to feel "high."

59. A 19-year-old college student goes to a party and is offered a substance to smoke. After doing so, he feels relaxed, at ease, and hungry. On examination, his conjunctiva are injected.

60. A 36-year-old woman decides to stop her daily intake of 5 cups of coffee per day. After 12 hours without the drug, she notices feeling tired, irritable, and has a headache.

61. A 45-year-old man decides to stop smoking "cold turkey." After 24 hours without a cigarette, he has an intense craving to smoke. He also notes that he is irritable and anxious.

62. A 25-year-old man is brought to the emergency room with a temperature of 102°F, blood pressure of 175/95 mm/Hg, and a heart rate of 120 beats/minute. He is noted to be disoriented, tremulous, and responding to auditory hallucinations. On examination, he has increased reflexes bilaterally. His friends tell the physician that he recently stopped using his regular drug of choice.

Evaluation, Assessment, and Diagnosis

Answers

1. The answer is b. (*Kaplan and Sadock, pp 275, 280.*) Circumstantiality indicates the loss of a goal-directed thought process: the patient brings in many irrelevant details and comments, but eventually will get back to the point. In loose associations, the thought process has also lost its goal-directedness; however, the patient never gets back to the original point and there is no clear connection between sentences. A neologism is a fabricated word made up by the patient, which is usually a combination of existing words. Perseveration, often associated with cognitive disorders, refers to a response that persists even after a new stimulus has been introduced—for example, a patient asked to repeat the phrase "no ifs, and, or buts" responds by saying, "no ifs, ifs, ifs, ifs." Flight of ideas is a disorder of thinking in which the patient expresses thoughts very rapidly, with constant shifting from one idea to another, though the ideas are often connected.

2. The answer is b. (*Kaplan and Sadock, p 1.*) A patient in this situation needs empathy above all else if a successful rapport is to be developed. Informing the patient that his problem is simple and easily fixed might eventually bring some relief to the patient, but if stated early in the interview process can sound condescending, as if the patient should not trouble the physician with such trivial things. Expressing compassion for the difficult situation the patient finds himself in is showing true empathy with the patient's current discomfort. Telling the patient that you are nervous about seeing new patients too could be seen as an expression of empathy with the patient, but may also make the patient feel dismayed, since he wants a confident and competent physician to treat him. Asking the patient why he is so unusually nervous will only make the patient *more* self-conscious, and it is *not* unusual for patients to be this nervous on a first visit to a psychiatrist (especially if they have never seen one before). Finally, getting right to the patient's complaint just ignores the uncomfortable feeling the patient has come in with, and this will not help the development of rapport (nor is it very observant of the psychiatrist).

3. The answer is e. *(Kaplan and Sadock, p 234.)* A neologism is either the use of a completely made up word or phrase, or the use of an existing word or phrase in an idiosyncratic manner. Clang associations are thoughts that come out in a rhyming pattern, whether or not the verbalized sentence means anything logically. Thought blocking is a sudden stoppage or "blocking" in the patient's pattern of thought, so much so that speech is disrupted as well. Tangentiality refers to a pattern of thought in which the patient answers a question with something that is related to the question, but does not answer it directly. For example, Question: "How are you feeling?" Answer: "This sofa is feeling particularly soft today." The patient's belief that the CIA is listening to his thoughts is an example of a paranoid delusion. A grandiose delusion involves believing that one is famous or of special importance. For example, "I know that the President would love to meet me because I have this talent." An auditory hallucination is the experience of hearing something that no one else can hear. For example, hearing a voice telling one to kill oneself. Labile affect is the rapid shifting of facial expression and behavior between two different emotional presentations. For example, a patient is laughing one minute, crying the next, and back to laughing shortly thereafter.

4. The answer is c. *(Kaplan and Sadock, pp 276, 278, 281-282.)* An illusion is the misperception or misinterpretation of a real sensory stimulus, as opposed to a hallucination, which is a false sensory perception unrelated to any real sensory stimulus. A delusion is a fixed, false belief that is unrelated to a patient's intelligence or cultural background. By definition, a delusion cannot be corrected with the use of logic or reasoning. Projection is a defense mechanism in which the patient reacts to an inner unacceptable impulse as if it were outside the self—for example, a paranoid patient reacts to others as if they were going to hurt him. This is because the patient's unacceptable hostile impulses are projected onto others, and the patient reacts as if the others have hostile impulses of their own toward the patient. Synesthesia is a sensation or hallucination caused by another sensation (eg, a visual sensation triggers the hallucination of an auditory sensation).

5. The answer is d. *(Kaplan and Sadock, p 235.)* Having a patient subtract 7s from 100 tests concentration. Orientation is evaluated by asking the patient whether he knows where he is, who he is, and what the date is. Immediate memory is tested by asking a patient to repeat a series of numbers immediately after you say them with no time delay. Fund of knowledge is tested by asking a patient to answer a question that an average adult would know the answer to, such as, "What is the body of water that lies off the east coast of New York?"

6. The answer is d. (*Moore and Jefferson, p 281.*) The diagnostic criteria for delirium include a disturbance of consciousness (ie, this woman's decreased arousal) and a change in cognition (ie, the inconsolable crying followed by the sudden appearance of paranoia in this woman). The disturbance must develop over a short period of time and tends to fluctuate over the course of a day. There also must be evidence that the disturbance is caused by the direct physiological consequence of a general medical condition, which must be assumed in this case. Since no prior history of a mental disorder was given, and the disturbance was not present immediately upon admission, it is unlikely that the patient has a major depression or is experiencing an acute manic episode. Since the patient's consciousness is waxing and waning, it is also unlikely that she is experiencing either a brief psychotic episode or an acute stress reaction.

7. The answer is b. (*Kaplan and Sadock, p 806.*) The essential feature of obsessive-compulsive personality disorder is a preoccupation with perfection, orderliness, and control. Individuals with this disorder lose the main point of an activity and miss deadlines because they pay too much attention to rules and details and are not satisfied with anything less than "perfection." As in other personality disorders, symptoms are ego-syntonic and create interpersonal, social, and occupational difficulties. Obsessive-compulsive disorder is differentiated from obsessive-compulsive personality disorder by the presence of obsessions and compulsions. In addition, patients with symptoms of obsessive-compulsive disorder view them as ego-dystonic. Patients with borderline personality disorder present with a history of pervasive instability of mood, relationships, and self-image beginning by early adulthood. Their behavior is often impulsive and self-damaging. Patients with bipolar disorder present with problems of mood stability; mood may be depressed for several weeks at a time, then euphoric. Patients with an anxiety disorder not otherwise specified present with anxiety as a main symptom, though they do not specifically fit any other, more specific anxiety disorder as per *DSM-IV-TR* (*Diagnostic and Statistical Manual, 4th edition*, text revision).

8. The answer is b. (*Jacobson and Jacobson, pp 85-91.*) The essential features of obsessive-compulsive disorder are obsessions (recurrent and persistent thoughts that are experienced as intrusive and inappropriate and that cause anxiety) and compulsions (repetitive behaviors that the person feels driven to perform). In this disorder, the patient's symptoms are ego-dystonic to him or her, unlike the person with an obsessive-compulsive personality disorder. Patients with attention-deficit hyperactivity disorder have problems with inattention, hyperactivity, and/or impulsivity. Patients with separation anxiety disorder worry about losing or harming major attachment figures and become anxious when separation from home or those major figures is anticipated. Patients with brief psychotic disorder show evidence of either delusions or hallucinations for a short period of time, usually after exposure to some external stressor.

9. The answer is c. *(Kaplan and Sadock, p 310.)* A global assessment of functioning between 51 and 60 denotes the presence of a moderate amount of symptoms. One can see mild symptomatology (eg, circumstantiality or occasional panic attacks) or this rating denotes moderate problems with social functioning (problems working, few friends, etc). The *DSM-IV* uses a multiaxial assessment system that evaluates patients along several lines. It contains five axes. Axis I consists of the psychiatric disorders that a patient may have, not including mental retardation or personality disorders. Axis II includes those two types of disorders. Axis III lists physical disorders (such as hypothyroidism) or other general medical conditions that the patient may have in addition to the psychiatric disorder, whether or not the physical disorder is related to the psychiatric disorder itself. Axis IV is used to list the psychosocial or environmental stressors that may have contributed to the development or exacerbation of the psychiatric disorder which is being addressed in Axis I or II. (For example, loss of significant other, divorce). Axis V, as noted above, is global assessment of functioning, considered a mixture of a patient's ability to function socially, occupationally, and psychologically.

10 to 13. The answers are 10-c, 11-f, 12-h, 13-b. *(Kaplan and Sadock, pp. 591, 795, 659, 500, 624.)* Patients with schizoid personality disorder are notable in that their symptoms (social isolation, inability to connect emotionally with others, tendency to daydream) are ego-syntonic—that is, they do not cause a problem for the patient and are not seen as such. These patients may have very few social connections, and unlike patients with avoidant personality disorder, they do not seem to miss the contact. Patients with schizotypal personality disorder, by contrast, are generally seen as odd, with eccentric (though not to the point of delusional) thoughts and beliefs. Patients with factitious disorder are trying to achieve the role of a person with an illness (usually physical) so that they may be cared for by the health-care system. This constitutes primary gain, in that there is usually nothing they are trying to avoid by adopting the sick role (as opposed to the secondary gain of malingering, whereby a patient might enter the hospital, eg, to avoid being arrested by the police). Patients often will have undergone a series of medical procedures, and it is not unusual to find a history of a family member (or the patient himself/herself) being involved in a medical field as a line of work.

Schizophreniform disorder is best thought of as a schizophrenia-like illness that simply has not been manifested for long enough to be called schizophrenia (6 months is the cutoff point between the two). Psychotic symptoms such as auditory or visual hallucinations are common, as is a premorbid history of being "weird" or a "loner." Generalized anxiety disorder is identified by the fact that the patient has multiple worries, not just one or two. For example, the anxious patient is not worried just about having an anxiety attack *or* about the health of her daughter *or* about the war in Iraq. She is worried about a number of different scenarios, and they are not all related.

14. The answer is b. (*Kaplan and Sadock, p 275.*) Patients who present with concrete thinking have lost the ability to form abstract concepts, such as metaphors, and focus instead on actual things and facts. Concrete thinking is the norm in children and is seen in cognitive disorders (mental retardation, dementia) and schizophrenia.

15. The answer is e. (*Kaplan and Sadock, p 906.*) The patient in this scenario has chronic issues with self-injury (which is confirmed by a psychiatrist that has been seeing her for a long period of time). She lives in a safe and supportive environment and is in ongoing outpatient care. The suicidal gesture occurred during an argument, and the gesture itself was not serious (ie, only 10 aspirin tablets were taken, and in front of the mother, so rescue was a certainty). Since the patient lives in a setting that is separate from her mother, it is likely that continued outpatient treatment and returning to the halfway home to live will be more beneficial to the patient than being admitted. Continued observation in an emergency room setting is unlikely to provide any benefit either.

16. The answer is a. (*Moore and Jefferson, pp 285, 346-347.*) Multiple cerebral infarcts cause a progressive dementia (usually described as stepwise), focal neurological signs, and often neuropsychiatric symptoms such as depression, mood lability (but usually not elated mood), and delusions.

Loose associations, catatonic posturing, and bizarre proverb interpretations occurring with affective symptoms are typical of schizoaffective disorder. In delirium, one would expect to see the waxing and waning of consciousness over time, including problems with orientation to person, place, and time. The patient does not have a mood disorder, because, although he is depressed over his loss of memory, he has no vegetative or other depressive symptoms other than mood.

17. The answer is c. (*Kaplan and Sadock, p 233.*) Mood is the pervasive and sustained emotion that the patient experiences. In this case, the patient states that she is sad and thus her mood might be described as such. A commonly used term to describe sad is dysphoric, as opposed to euphoric (extremely happy) or euthymic (normal state of mood—neither high nor low). Affect is the patient's present emotionally responsive state, and it is inferred by the patient's facial expression, speech, and body language. Affect may or may not be congruent with mood. For example, a patient who states that he is sad, but is laughing and jovial throughout the interview might be said to have a dysphoric mood with an incongruent affect. The patient in the vignette also has a constricted affect, in that during the interview she appears sad all the time. She never displays anything but this emotion and thus is constricted to the low end (depressed end) of the emotional range.

18. The answer is c. (*Moore and Jefferson, pp 12-14.*) The diagnosis of mental retardation is made after a history, IQ test, and measures of adaptive functioning indicate that the behavior is significantly below the level expected. An EEG is rarely helpful except for those patients who have grand mal seizures. While the presence of temper tantrums in a young child might be a sign of a psychiatric disorder such as a major depression, the Beck depression test is designed for use patients of 13 years of age and above. In addition, elements of the history such as the child's continued enjoyment of playing with her toys makes this diagnosis less likely. Metabolic disorders can cause mental retardation, but a CBC would be unlikely to pick this up. A lumbar puncture would be helpful only if the physician believed these symptoms to be secondary to an infectious process—unlikely, given the time course.

19. The answer is b. (*Kaplan and Sadock, p 911.*) Alcohol intoxication and an overt stressor (impending breakup with the girlfriend) are both predictors of violence. Demographically, males from the ages of 15 to 24 are more likely to commit violent acts, and this patient is outside that age range. Also, those with low socioeconomic statuses and few social supports are more likely to commit violent acts. While verbal threats of physical violence do increase the risk of subsequent physical violence, the age difference of the couple in question has no bearing on the prediction of violence.

20. The answer is a. *(Kaplan and Sadock, p 912.)* The first order of business with a physically violent patient is to ensure the safety of the patient and the caregivers. Since this patient has already been physically violent, it is not the time to reason with the patient verbally, or offer medication orally. The patient should be put immediately in full leather restraints (not soft restraints). Since medical students and residents are rarely fully trained in the safe restraint of a violent patient, this is better done by those who are trained, if at all possible.

21. The answer is a. *(Kaplan and Sadock, p 912.)* The patient is still struggling and out of control while in restraints, so the next action that should be taken is to sedate him. This is best achieved in an emergency room setting with the IM combination of haloperidol and lorazepam (which both decreases the dose of antipsychotic necessary and protects against dystonic reactions). An IV would be extremely difficult to start with a struggling patient and valium should never be given IV push at any rate. While drawing blood for additional toxicology screens is probably a good idea, the first priority should be to control this patient's behavior before he injures himself.

22. The answer is c. *(Jacobson and Jacobson, p 500.)* Countertransference is the name given to the analyst's or psychotherapist's transference response to the patient. As with patients' transference, the particular form the countertransference takes depends on the therapist's past experiences, relationships, and unresolved conflicts. As with transference, countertransference is not limited to the patient–therapist relationship, but may be present in any relationship. By analyzing his or her countertransference toward the patient, the therapist may acquire useful insight into the patient's dynamics and his or her own. Consequently, even negative countertransference feelings can be helpful tools in the psychotherapy process. Reaction formation, projection, and identification with the aggressor are unconscious defense mechanisms. An illusion is a perceptual misinterpretation of a real stimulus.

23. The answer is d. *(Kaplan and Sadock, pp 323-328.)* The patient's persecutory delusions and disorganized thinking could suggest a psychotic disorder such as schizophrenia or brief reactive psychosis, but fluctuations in consciousness and disorientation are typically found in delirium. Memory, language, and sleep–wake cycle disturbances are also typical of delirium. Delusions, hallucinations, illusions, and misperceptions are also common. The causes of delirium are many and include metabolic encephalopathies (including fever and hypoxia, as in the patient in the question), intoxications with drugs and poisons, withdrawal syndromes, head trauma, epilepsy, neoplasms, vascular disorders, allergic reactions, and injuries caused by physical agents (heat, cold, radiation).

24. The answer is d. (*Jacobson and Jacobson, pp 400-406.*) The patient has HIV-associated dementia, a disorder caused by the direct toxic effect of HIV on the brain. A CD4 count below 200 is usually associated with HIV dementia, since this disorder typically occurs in the more advanced stages of AIDS. More rarely, cognitive impairments may be the first manifestation of HIV infection.

25. The answer is d. (*Moore and Jefferson, pp 253-255.*) Individuals with borderline personality disorder characteristically form intense but very unstable relationships. Since they tend to perceive themselves and others as either totally bad or perfectly good, borderline individuals either idealize or devalue any person who occupies a significant place in their lives. Usually these perceptions do not last, and the person idealized one day can be seen as completely negative the next day. This inability to see people as integrated wholes of both good and bad aspects, but rather to put them in the "all" or "none" category, is called splitting.

26. The answer is b. (*Moore and Jefferson, p 179.*) Conversion disorder is characterized by the sudden appearance of often dramatic neurological symptoms that are not associated with the usual diagnostic signs and test results expected for the symptoms being presented. Conversion disorder occurs in the context of a psychosocial stressor or an insoluble interpersonal or intrapsychic conflict. The psychological distress is not consciously acknowledged, but it is expressed through a metaphorical body dysfunction. In this example, the man who is torn between his duty to his mother and his intense anger at her resolved his impulse to hit her by developing a physical paralysis of his right arm.

27. The answer is e. (*Moore and Jefferson, pp 11, 165-167.*) A social phobia is a persistent and overwhelming fear of humiliation or embarrassment in social or performance situations. This leads to high levels of distress and avoidance of those situations. Often, physical symptoms of anxiety such as blushing, trembling, sweating, or tachycardia are triggered when the patient feels under evaluation or scrutiny.

28. The answer is c. *(Kaplan and Sadock, p 175.)* Sensitivity is defined as the number of true positives divided by the sum of the number of true positives and false negatives. It is the proportion of patients with the condition in question that the test can detect. Thus, if the sensitivity is only 64%, the number of false negatives will most likely be unacceptably high.

29. The answer is d. *(Jacobson and Jacobson, p 11.)* Perseveration and circumstantiality are forms of thought disorder. In perseveration, the patient displays an inability to change the topic or gives the same response to different questions. Circumstantiality is a disturbance in which the patient digresses into unnecessary details before communicating the central idea. The capacity to generalize and to formulate concepts is called abstract thinking. The inability to abstract is called concreteness and is seen in organic disorders and sometimes in schizophrenia. Abstract thinking is commonly assessed by testing similarities, differences, and the meaning of proverbs. Negative symptoms include amotivation, apathy, and social withdrawal. These symptoms are often seen in schizophrenia.

30. The answer is c. *(Moore and Jefferson, p 9.)* Tangentiality, circumstantiality, flight of ideas, and looseness of associations are forms of thought disorder. Circumstantiality is a disturbance in which the patient digresses into unnecessary details before communicating the central idea. Tangentiality is present when the patient wanders and digresses to unnecessary details and the substance of the idea is never communicated. In flight of ideas, there are rapid, continuous verbalizations or plays on words that produce constant shifting from one idea to another. Ideas tend to be connected. In looseness of associations, the flow of thought is disconnected—ideas shift from one subject to another in a completely unrelated way.

31. The answer is b. *(Moore and Jefferson, p 9.)* In thought blocking, the patient suddenly stops talking, usually in the middle of a sentence, and cannot complete his or her thoughts. Affect is said to be incongruent when what is observed by the examiner (affect) does not match the subjective statement of how the patient feels (mood). Perseveration is a form of thought disorder in which the patient displays an inability to change the topic or gives the same response to different questions. Thought insertion refers to the patient's idea that some thought content is being inserted directly into the patient's mind.

32. The answer is e. (*Moore and Jefferson, p 198.*) Derealization is the subjective sense that the environment is strange or unreal, as if reality had been changed. Perception is a physical sensation given a meaning or the integration of sensory stimuli to form an image or impression; in dulled perception, this capacity is diminished. Retardation of thought refers to the slowing of thought processes that may be seen in major depression. Response time to questions may be increased. Depersonalization refers to feeling that one is falling apart or not one's self, that one's self is unreal or detached.

33. The answer is b. (*Kaplan and Sadock, p 279.*) Magical thinking is a form of thinking similar to that of preoperational-phase children (from work by Jean Piaget) in which thoughts and ideas are believed to have special powers (eg, to cause or stop outside events). In thought broadcasting, the patient senses that his or her thoughts are being stolen, are leaking out of the mind, or are being sent out to others across radio or television. Echolalia refers to the repetition of the examiner's words or phrases by the patient. Nihilism is the belief that oneself, others, or the world are either nonexistent or are coming to an end. An obsession is the ego-dystonic persistence of a thought or feeling that cannot be eliminated from consciousness voluntarily.

34 to 37. The answers are 34-b, 35-a, 36-c, 37-c. (*Kaplan and Sadock, p 662.*) Malingering is the intentional production of medical or psychiatric complaints in the hope of some secondary gain (eg, getting out of work or prison). A factitious disorder, in contrast, is the intentional production of medical or psychiatric complaints to get the patient some kind of primary gain (usually getting to fulfill the cared-for role of a patient). Both somatization and conversion disorders are complaints that are unconsciously and unintentionally produced.

38. The answer is d. (*Moore and Jefferson, pp 4, 132-133, 186-187; Kaplan and Sadock, p 276.*) Echopraxia is the mimicking of the examiner's body posture and movements by the patient. This can be seen in chronic schizophrenia. Folie à deux is a shared psychotic (delusional) belief held by two people. Dereistic thinking is a thought activity not concordant with logic or experience. Echolalia refers to the repetition of the examiner's words or phrases by the patient. Fugue is the taking on of a new identity with no memory of the old one. It often involves travel to a new environment.

39 to 41. The answers are 39-c, 40-e, 41-b. *(Jacobson and Jacobson, pp 18-99.)* Axis I is the place to record all primary psychiatric disorders other than mental retardation or personality disorders, which are recorded on Axis II. Axis III is where medical conditions of all kinds, whether or not they are related to the primary psychiatric diagnosis, are recorded. Axis IV is the place to record stressors that are occurring in the patient's life—including social, legal, or financial situations. Axis V records the global assessment of functioning, on a scale of 0 to 100.

42 to 45. The answers are 42-b, 43-c, 44-d, 45-a. *(Ebert et al, pp 417, 521, 580-592.)* Conduct disorder is usually diagnosed in adolescence, and consists of a repetitive and persistent pattern of behavior in which the basic rights of others, and appropriate social norms, are violated. Categories of criteria include: aggression to people or animals; destruction of property; deceitfulness or theft; or serious violations of rules (staying out all night, running away from home, truancy from school). Three of the criteria must be met in the past 12 months, with at least one criterion present in the last year.

Antisocial personality disorder is only diagnosed in an individual of at least 18 years of age, though there must be evidence of a conduct disorder previously. This is a pervasive pattern of disregard and violation of the rights of others occurring since age 15. Symptoms include: failure to conform to societal norms, deceitfulness, impulsivity, irritability and aggressiveness, reckless disregard for the safety of self or others, consistent irresponsibility, and a lack of remorse.

Malingering is a deliberate disease simulation with a specific, secondary gain in mind (to get drugs, to avoid being caught by the police). Malingering may include the deliberate production of disease or the exaggeration, elaboration, or false report of symptoms.

Oppositional defiant disorder is not as dysfunctional as conduct disorder, in that the main behavior is that of defiance: losing temper, arguing with adults, defying rules, annoying people, blaming others for mistakes, angry, resentful, or spiteful. (See conduct disorder answer above for the more serious behavior which constitutes that diagnosis.)

46 to 52. The answers are 46-g, 47-b, 48-f, 49-a, 50-e, 51-c, 52-d. *(Ebert et al, pp 679-690.)* Malignant hyperthermia may occur as a result of the administration of neuromuscular junction blockers (succinylcholine, halathone, etc). It results in symptoms of hyperthermia, muscle rigidity, arrhythmias, hypotension, rhabdomyolysis, and disseminated intravascular coagulation. As noted in the vignette, hypersensitivity to these kinds of medications run in families.

Neuroleptic malignant syndrome is a serious and potentially lethal problem brought about by the use of neuroleptics. Three sets of symptoms appear rapidly: alteration in level of consciousness, autonomic instability (hyperthermia, tachycardia, labile hypertension, and tachypnea) and "lead pipe" muscle rigidity. Elevated creatinine phosphokinase level and leukocytosis are common findings. The syndrome can appear at any time, not just after the initiation of an antipsychotic.

Thyrotoxicosis (or thyroid storm) is a rare but severe complication of hyperthyroidism, which may occur when a thyrotoxic patient becomes very sick or physically stressed. Its symptoms can include: an increase in body temperature to over 40°C (104°F), tachycardia, arrhythmia, vomiting, diarrhea, dehydration, coma, and death. Thyroid storm requires emergency treatment and hospitalization.

Anticholinergic syndrome is most often seen in vulnerable populations (as in the elderly) who may have been given (or have taken) multiple medications with anticholinergic properties. Anticholinergic syndrome is characterized by blurry vision, dry mouth, and constipation, as well as confusion and delirium in severe cases.

Serotonin syndrome occurs when plasma serotonin concentrations reach toxic levels. This can occur with concurrent administration of an SSRI with an MAOI, l-tryptophan, or lithium. The condition has the following symptoms (in order of appearance as the condition worsens): diarrhea; restlessness; extreme agitation, hyperreflexia, and autonomic instability; myoclonus; seizures, hyperthermia, uncontrollable shivering, and rigidity; delirium, coma, status epilepticus, and death.

Acute dystonic reactions include facial grimacing and torticollis. These are extrapyramidal motor disturbances consisting of slow, sustained contractions of the axial or appendicular muscles. One movement often predominates, leading to relatively sustained postural deviations. These reactions are seen on occasion with the initiation of antipsychotic drug therapy.

Akathisia is a subjective feeling of motor restlessness manifested by the patient's need to be in almost constant movement. This may be seen as an extrapyramidal side effect after the initiation of antipsychotic therapy.

It must be carefully delineated from psychotic agitation, since treating the latter with antipsychotics can make the akathisia much worse.

53 to 62. The answers are 53-d, 54-i, 55-a, 56-e, 57-j, 58-f, 59-g, 60-b, 61-h, 62-c *(Kaplan and Sadock, p 119.)* The patient in vignette 53 has suffered a seizure. This disorder is characterized on EEG interictally by epileptiform discharges.

The patient in vignette 54 has hepatic encephalopathy. Approximately one-half of patients with triphasic waves on EEG have hepatic encephalopathy.

The patient in vignette 55 has a general toxic encephalopathy (in this case due to an electrolyte imbalance). A diffuse slowing of background rhythms is often present in patients with diffuse encephalopathies of diverse causes.

The patient in vignette 56 has had a stroke. Periodic lateralizing epileptiform discharges suggest the presence of an acute destructive cerebral lesion and are associated with focal neurological findings.

The patient in vignette 57 has Creutzfeldt-Jakob disease. Ninety percent of patients with this disease have generalized periodic sharp waves seen on EEG.

The patient in vignette 58 has opioid intoxication. Characteristic findings on EEG include decreased alpha activity and increased voltage of theta and delta waves. In overdose with this drug, slow waves may be seen on EEG.

The patient in vignette 59 has used marijuana. This drug increased alpha activity in the frontal area of the brain, but overall slows alpha activity.

The patient in vignette 60 is in caffeine withdrawal. There is an increase in amplitude or voltage of theta activity on EEG with this condition.

The patient in vignette 61 is in nicotine withdrawal. There is a marked decrease in alpha activity seen on the EEG during the withdrawal period.

The patient in vignette 62 is undergoing barbiturate withdrawal. In withdrawal states, EEG shows generalized paroxysmal activity and spike discharges.

Human Behavior: Theories of Personality and Development

Questions

63. A 6-month-old male infant is noted by his mother to be difficult to care for. He is very difficult to feed or soothe, and often responds to cuddling by crying and becoming rigid in his mother's arms. Physical examination and laboratory work are all entirely normal. Which of the following psychiatric disorders is this infant at a higher risk to display in his early school years?

a. Conduct disorder
b. Childhood schizophrenia
c. Separation anxiety disorder
d. Antisocial personality disorder
e. Pica

64. A 2-year-old girl is being toilet trained by her parents. Each time she soils her diaper, she is told that she is a very bad girl and she is punished by having a toy taken away. When she uses the toilet appropriately, she is not praised by her parents. Which of the following sequelae is the child most likely to experience as a result of this kind of parental behavior?

a. A basic sense of mistrust
b. Shame and self-doubt
c. Guilt
d. Stagnation of her development
e. An absence of intimacy as an adult

65. A 20-month-old boy loves running around and exploring the environment, but every few minutes he returns to his mother to check on her and solicit a quick hug. Which of the following best describes this behavior, according to Margaret Mahler?

a. Depressive position
b. Secure attachment
c. Insecure attachment
d. Rapprochement
e. Autonomy, versus shame and doubt

66. A woman brings her 18-month-old child to the psychiatrist, worried that he is not developing normally. The psychiatrist tests the child in three arenas, motor & sensory behavior, adaptive behavior, and personal & social behavior and finds the following (the highest level of skill the child achieves during these tests is outlined):

Motor & Sensory Behavior	Adaptive Behavior	Personal & Social Behavior
Can hurl ball and walk up stairs with one hand held	Can build a tower of 3 to 4 cubes; scribbles spontaneously	Has separation anxiety when taken away from his mother; holds own bottle

Which of the following best describes his current state of development?

a. Accelerated development in all three areas
b. Accelerated motor & sensory behavior, normal adaptive behavior, and personal & social behavior
c. Normal motor & sensory and adaptive behavior, delayed personal & social behavior
d. Delayed motor & sensory and adaptive behavior, normal personal & social behavior
e. Delayed development in all three areas

67. A 2-year-old child carries around an old, tattered blanket wherever he goes. When he is sad or upset, he calms himself by hugging and stroking his blanket. He also needs it to settle down before sleep. For this child, which of the following does his blanket best represent?

a. Fetish
b. Obsession
c. Transitional object
d. Transference object
e. Imaginary friend

68. A 4-year-old child is brought to the psychiatrist by her mother. Although the child is developing normally, she is scheduled to have her tonsils removed. The mother wishes to make this operation as smooth and atraumatic as possible. Using Piaget's theory, what should the psychiatrist tell the mother about how this upcoming event should be explained to the child?

a. No explanation will be helpful; the mother should try to stay with the child at all times.
b. No explanation need be given, but the child should be asked what questions she has about the upcoming event and those questions should be answered.
c. Verbal explanations will not be helpful. The upcoming event should be role played with the child through the use of dolls and toys.
d. A simplified verbal explanation should be given to the child.
e. A verbal explanation of the operation should be given, with all the terms the child will hear in the hospital used. The child should be engaged in a question and answer session afterward.

69. A 32-year-old woman is given the news by her physician that she has breast cancer and will need surgery, followed by chemotherapy. She returns home after the appointment, and her husband asks how the visit went. She tells him that "everything was fine." For the rest of the evening, she behaves as if there had been no bad news given to her. In fact, she appears to be in good spirits. Which of the following defense mechanisms is likely being employed by this woman?

a. Denial
b. Projection
c. Sublimation
d. Reaction formation
e. Altruism

70. A 3-year-old boy stands on one side of a large sculpture and is asked to describe what he sees. When asked to describe what a person on the other side of the sculpture sees, the child answers that the other person sees just what he does. Which of the following theories uses the concept described above?

a. Psychosexual development
b. Moral development
c. Cognitive development
d. Social development
e. Autism

71. A 70-year-old woman is admitted to the hospital after a fall in which she broke her left hip. She is a difficult patient during her rehabilitation phase, passively resisting attempts to get her up and walking, contending that it does not matter whether she regains her capacity to walk on her own since she is so advanced in age. She states that while she is fearful of dying, she feels disgust at her own body because it is "falling apart." Which of the following Eriksonian stages is this patient most likely working through?

a. Integrity versus despair
b. Intimacy versus isolation
c. Generativity versus stagnation
d. Identity versus role diffusion
e. Industry versus inferiority

72. A young woman with a history of childhood neglect feels suddenly worthless and devastated when her supervisor makes a mildly negative comment about her work performance. According to Heinz Kohut, which of the following explanations accounts for her hypersensitivity to criticism?

a. An unresolved oedipal complex due to her parents' divorce when the woman was 4 years old
b. An inability to make stable commitments to others
c. A punitive superego due to harsh and critical parents
d. A fragmented sense of self due to the empathic failure of her parents
e. Autistic traits

73. A 16-year-old boy is diagnosed with osteosarcoma. Surgery and chemotherapy are not successful as treatments, and it is apparent that the child will die from his disease. The child, rather than focusing on his death, seems more concerned with the fact that he has lost all his hair from the chemotherapy. He is difficult to work with in the hospital, as he insists on seeing visitors only when he chooses to and wants to work with only his favorite nurses. Which of the following is the best explanation for his behavior?

a. He is regressing under the stress of his terminal illness.
b. He is an adolescent and these responses are quite typical for the age group.
c. He has developed a major depression.
d. He is in denial of his impending death.
e. He is having a cognitive disturbance secondary to brain metastases.

74. A 23-year-old man impulsively steals a pack of gum at a convenience store. He has never stolen anything previously, and almost immediately upon exiting the store with the gum, he begins to feel extremely guilty. Which of the following concepts introduced by Freud is most likely responsible for this man's emotional response to his theft?

a. Id
b. Ego
c. Superego
d. Preconscious function
e. Conscious function

75. A 20-month-old girl is admitted to a pediatric ward because she weighs only 15 lb. An extensive medical work-up does not reveal any organic cause for the child's failure to thrive. The child is listless and apathetic and does not smile. The parents rarely come to visit, and when they do, they do not pick the child up and do not play or interact with her. Which of the following statements best explains this scenario?

a. Lack of adequate emotional nurturance causes depression and failure to thrive in infants.
b. Neglected infants fail to thrive but do not have the intrapsychic structures necessary for experiencing depression.
c. Infants reared in institutions are likely to become autistic.
d. Neglected infants are at higher risk for developing schizophrenia.
d. Environmental variables have little impact on the health of infants as long as enough food is provided.

76. A 25-year-old woman sees a psychiatrist for a chief complaint of having a depressed mood for her "entire life." She begins psychotherapy and sees the physician once per week. After 3 months of therapy, she tells the psychiatrist that she is very afraid of him because he is "so angry all the time." She behaves as if this is true and that the psychiatrist will explode with rage at any minute. The psychiatrist is not normally seen as an angry person and is unaware of any anger toward the patient. Which of the following defense mechanisms is this patient likely displaying?

a. Distortion
b. Blocking
c. Isolation
d. Projection
e. Dissociation

77. A healthy 9-month-old girl is brought to her pediatrician by her concerned parents. Previously very friendly with everyone, she now bursts into tears when she is approached by an unfamiliar adult. Which of the following best describes this child's behavior?

a. Separation anxiety
b. Insecure attachment
c. Simple phobia
d. Depressive position
e. Stranger anxiety

78. According to Sigmund Freud, which of the following best describes primary processes?

a. Typically conscious
b. Nonlogical and primitive
c. Absent during dreaming
d. Characteristic of the neuroses
e. Rational and well-organized

79. A woman has a verbal altercation with her boss at work. She meekly accepts his harsh words. That night, she picks a fight with her husband. Which of the following defense mechanisms is being used by this woman?

a. Displacement
b. Acting out
c. Reaction formation
d. Projection
e. Sublimation

80. A 24-year-old woman lives with her mother, whom she intensely dislikes. She feels embarrassed by this, and compensates by hovering over her mother, attending to her every need. Which of the following defense mechanisms is being used by this woman?

a. Displacement
b. Acting out
c. Reaction formation
d. Rationalization
e. Sublimation

81. A writer of mystery novels, who has never had legal problems, jokes about his "dark side" and his hidden fantasies about leading an exciting life of crime. Which of the following defense mechanisms is being used by this man?

a. Anticipation
b. Sublimation
c. Identification with the aggressor
d. Introjection
e. Distortion

82. A 35-year-old man is being seen by his psychiatrist for depressed mood. The patient is irritated at his therapist for pushing him on several issues in the last session. The patient does not show up or call for his next session. Which of the following defense mechanisms is this patient displaying?

a. Introjection
b. Sublimation
c. Identification with the aggressor
d. Acting out
e. Intellectualization

83. A 45-year-old man accidentally crashes his car into another vehicle. He feels extremely guilty, and in order to avoid these feelings of self-reproach, he explains in meticulous detail to anyone listening all of the steps leading up to his accident. Which of the following defense mechanisms is this patient displaying?

a. Sublimation
b. Repression
c. Intellectualization
d. Acting out
e. Rationalization

84. A 45-year-old woman is admitted to the hospital after her son finds her unconscious at home. She is treated for diabetic ketoacidosis and her recovery is a difficult one, necessitating that she stay in the hospital for 5 days. During this period of time, she is often angry, irrational, and demanding, all of which are not her usual modes of behavior or thinking, according to her husband. What is the most likely explanation for the change in this woman's behavior?

a. The fluid shifts that are occurring during the stabilization of her diabetes are causing an organic mood disorder.
b. Her fear of a newly diagnosed illness is causing her to dissociate.
c. The stress of her illness and hospital stay is causing her to regress.
d. She is delirious secondary to brain damage from her period of unconsciousness.
e. A previously unrecognized personality disorder is coming to the fore.

85. A 38-year-old woman comes to a psychiatrist for help with the management of her obsessive-compulsive disorder. She describes an impulse that she has frequently and that frightens her. This impulse is to murder her three children by blowing out the pilot light on her home's heater, thereby blowing up her house. As a result, she finds herself checking on the pilot light in her home at least 30 times a day. She carries a book of matches with her during these checks so that she might immediately relight the pilot light if she finds that it is out. Which of the following defense mechanisms does this act of checking the pilot light represent?

a. Reaction formation
b. Isolation
c. Undoing
d. Denial
e. Altruism

86. A 20-month-old male infant is placed in an emergency department of children and family services shelter after his mother is hospitalized as the result of a car accident. Three days after the separation, the child spends almost every waking moment crying and calling and searching for his mother. The fourth day after the separation, when the mother of the child comes to the shelter to reclaim her child, he adamantly rejects her offers of affection, instead clinging to the nurse's aide who has been his caretaker. Which of the following terms most accurately describes this infant's reactions to a forced separation?

a. Protest
b. Despair
c. Detachment
d. Denial
e. Acting out

87. A 17-month-old girl is playing with her mother. Her mother hides a large red ball from the child and encourages her to find it. The girl looks under several pieces of furniture and finally finds the ball hidden behind the couch. The mother enjoys this game, because 2 months previously, if she had tried to play this game, the child simply would not have been able to understand that once the ball was out of sight it still existed. This advance in cognitive ability is most accurately described by which of the following terms?

a. Transitional object
b. Preoperational thought
c. Parallel play
d. Concrete operations
e. Object permanence

88. A 5-year-old girl loves her father's attention and becomes irritated with her mother when her mother kisses her father. The child tells her father she wants to marry him when she grows up. Which Freudian theory best describes the developmental stages this child is in?

a. Oral
b. Anal
c. Phallic
d. Oedipal
e. Latency

89. Which of Freud's theories deals with a model of the mind divided into three regions—conscious, unconscious, and preconscious?

a. Parapraxes
b. Infantile sexuality
c. Structural
d. Topographic
e. Primary process

90. Which of the following is the single most significant developmental event of middle childhood (typically defined as between the ages of 6 and 12)?

a. The onset of puberty
b. Going to school
c. The development of an overt interest in the opposite sex
d. The consolidation of personality
e. A growing concern with cultural values and ideologies

Human Behavior: Theories of Personality and Development

Answers

63. The answer is a. (*Kaplan and Sadock, p 27.*) This infant has what has been characterized as a "difficult" temperament. Infants with this temperament, as opposed to "easy" temperaments, have been shown to be at risk in the early school years for conduct problems. This correlation, although somewhat weaker, is also present through adolescence. The diagnosis of antisocial personality disorder is not given to patients under the age of 18. There is no evidence for any of the other psychiatric disorders as listed.

64. The answer is b. (*Kaplan and Sadock, p 209.*) Children from the ages of approximately 1 to 3 are in the Eriksonian stage of autonomy versus shame and doubt. Children who are shamed by their caregivers—as in this example of the child who does not go to the toilet but, rather, soils her diapers—are more likely to develop shame and self-doubt rather than functioning autonomously with a sense of pride and self-confidence. The other options listed in this question are negative sequelae that can occur in other phases of the Eriksonian stages of the life cycle: basic trust versus mistrust (birth to 1 year), initiative versus guilt (3 to 5 years), intimacy versus isolation (21 to 40 years), and generativity versus stagnation (40 to 65 years).

65. The answer is d. (*Kaplan and Sadock, p 29.*) Margaret Mahler made her contributions to the psychoanalytic movement called ego psychology through her theories on early infantile development. On the basis of her observations of normal and pathological mother–child interactions, Mahler identified three phases of infant development. The autistic phase occurs during the first 2 months of life, when the child spends a good part of his or her day asleep and has little interest in interpersonal relationships. From 2 to 6 months, the child enters symbiosis, a stage characterized by psychological fusion or lack of differentiation between mother and child. Margaret

Mahler is best known, however, for her research on the third phase, called separation-individuation. During this phase, which occurs between 6 and 36 months, the child develops a concept of him- or herself as different and separated from the mother. During the same period, the infant gradually develops an internal, stable representation (introjection) of the mother, which includes both her positive and her negative aspects. The separation-individuation phase is divided into four subphases: differentiation, between 6 and 10 months, refers to the child's initial awareness that the mother is a separate person; practicing, between 10 and 16 months, is characterized by the child's enthusiastic exploration of the environment as a result of his or her newly acquired mobility; rapprochement, between 16 and 24 months, refers to a period characterized by a need to know where the mother is and frequent "refueling," triggered by the child's new awareness that independence also makes him or her vulnerable; the fourth subphase, object constancy, takes place during the third year of life and refers to the integration of the good and bad aspects of the internalized images of both the mother and the child's self. According to ego psychology theory, object constancy is necessary for the later development of stable and mature interpersonal relationships.

In Melanie Klein's theory of infantile psychological development, the depressive position refers to the period during which the infant realizes that the "bad mother" who frustrates the child's wishes and the "good mother" who nurtures him or her are the same person, and the child worries that rage at the "bad mother" may also destroy the good. Autonomy versus shame and doubt is one of the eight stages of psychosocial development described by Erikson and corresponds in age to the period of Mahler's separation-individuation.

66. The answer is c. (*Kaplan and Sadock, p 23.*) While an 18-month-old child is "on track" in the areas of motor & sensory behavior and adaptive behavior if he can do the tasks listed in the question, he is behind in the areas of personal and social behavior. At 18 months of age, a child in this last area of behavior should be able to feed himself (at least in part), pull a toy on a string, carry around a favorite doll or imitate (albeit with some delay) some behavioral patterns he sees. This child is at approximately the 40th week (10th month) of age development for personal and social behavior.

67. The answer is c. (*Kaplan and Sadock, p 226.*) D. W. Winnicott, a British pediatrician with a keen interest in psychoanalysis, focused his attention on the early mother–child relationship. In his view, the child is able to develop a separate and stable identity only if the child's needs are met by his or her mother's empathic anticipation. Winnicott calls the positive environment so created by the mother the holding environment. According to Winnicott, mothers do not have to be perfect in order to fulfill their roles, but they have to be good enough to provide the infant with a sufficient amount of comfort and constancy. Winnicott also coined the term transitional object, usually a toy or a blanket, which represents a comforting substitute for the primary caregiver. Thanks to a transitional object, the child can tolerate separation from the mother without excessive anxiety.

68. The answer is c. (*Kaplan and Sadock, p 136.*) This 4-year-old child is developing normally, placing her at the preoperational stage of development according to Piaget. Such children do not understand concepts and are unable to abstract, thus they benefit from role-playing what will occur in the hospital more than any kind of verbal descriptions.

69. The answer is a. (*Kaplan and Sadock, p 206.*) This patient is in denial, a defense mechanism in which the conscious awareness of a painful reality (in this case, the bad news about her breast cancer) is abolished. This patient is not pretending that her doctor's visit was uneventful; she actually consciously believes that her doctor's visit was fine. Projection is the act of perceiving and acting as if unacceptable internal impulses (which are unconscious) are coming from the external realm. For example, a patient with very aggressive impulses, which are unacceptable to him, begins acting as if the person in the room with him were being aggressive toward him. Sublimation is the act of transforming unacceptable social impulses into acceptable ones, in order to achieve impulse gratification. For example, a man with strong homicidal impulses writes extremely graphic but successful horror novels as a way to channel those unacceptable feelings into something socially appropriate. Reaction formation is the transformation of an unacceptable impulse into its opposite. For example, a woman who has feelings of hate and disgust toward another finds these impulses unacceptable, so instead she behaves as if this other person is a good friend. Altruism uses service to others as a way of getting one's instincts gratified.

70. The answer is c. (*Kaplan and Sadock, p 134.*) Egocentrism refers to the young child's inability to see things from another's point of view. Egocentrism is described by Jean Piaget as part of the preoperational stage of cognitive development, which occurs between 2 and 5 to 7 years of age.

71. The answer is a. *(Kaplan and Sadock, pp 207-213.)* Erik Erikson's theory of psychosocial development centers around eight stages of ego development that take place during the life cycle. Each stage represents a turning point in which physical, cognitive, social, and emotional changes trigger an internal crisis whose resolution results either in psychological growth or regression.

Erikson Stage	Age at Which it Occurs	Hallmarks of the Stage
Trust vs mistrust	Birth to 18 months	If the infant's needs are promptly and empathically met, the infant learns to see the world as a benign and nurturing place
Autonomy vs shame and doubt	18 months to 3 years	This stage corresponds to Freud's anal stage and Mahler's separation-individuation stage. During this period, if allowed to experiment with his or her new motility and curiosity about the environment, and if at the same time he or she is provided with enough nurturance, the child acquires a healthy self-esteem and sense of autonomy
Initiative vs guilt	3 to 5 years	The child expands his or her explorations of the outside world and has omnipotent fantasies about his or her own powers. During this stage, in a good psychosocial environment, the child develops a capacity for self-reflection, manifested by the child's feeling guilty when rules are broken, without losing enthusiasm for independent exploration
Industry vs inferiority	5 to 13 years	Equivalent to Freud's period of latency. The child's psychological growth depends on his or her opportunity to learn new skills and take pride in accomplishments
Identity vs role confusion	13 to 21 years	If this stage is mastered successfully, the young individual enters adulthood with a solid sense of identity, knowing his or her role in society

(Continued)

Intimacy vs isolation	21 to 40 years	Adult developmental task of learning to make and honor commitments to other people and to ideas
Generativity vs stagnations	40 to 60 years	The focus of the individual starts shifting from personal accomplishments and needs to a concern for the rest of society and the nurturing of the next generation
Integrity vs despair	60 to death	The main developmental task is accepting life as it is, without desire to change the past or change others. When this stage is mastered, the individual acquires the wisdom necessary to face the inevitability of death with equanimity and without dread

72. The answer is d. (*Kaplan and Sadock, pp 219-220.*) According to Kohut, empathic validation from caregivers is essential for the development of an integrated sense of self. People who have been neglected or abused or have received suboptimal parenting grow up with a very fragile sense of self and an easily shaken self-esteem. These individuals, like the woman in the question, cannot maintain a positive image of themselves when exposed to criticism or rejection and experience a devastating sense of worthlessness and fragmentation.

73. The answer is b. (*Kaplan and Sadock, p 39.*) This unfortunate adolescent is reacting to his impending death in a characteristic way for one of his age group. Adolescents are often preoccupied with their body image and control of their environment, even when they are not ill. These issues do not disappear for a terminally ill teen, but the focus on them may seem trivial to adults. Likewise, the need to assert their independence may be shown by their choosing which visitors they will see, which health-care staff members they will work with, and whom they will talk to on any given day.

74. The answer is c. (*Kaplan and Sadock, pp 199-200.*) In his structural theory of the mind, Freud divided the psychic apparatus into three agencies: the id, which contains the instinctual drives; the ego, whose function is to find an equilibrium between gratification of the instinctual drives and the rules of society (and the demands of the superego); and the superego, the agency that contains the internalized parental and societal rules and dictates to the ego what is not to be done. Guilt is the consequence of transgressing the superego's prohibitions. Preconscious and conscious functions are dimensions of the ego. Logical and abstract thinking as well as verbal expression come from these functions.

75. The answer is a. *(Kaplan and Sadock, pp 137-140.)* Although the relationships between emotional deprivation and failure to thrive are complex, the fact that children who are emotionally deprived do not grow well even when an adequate amount of food is available, is well proven. Renée Spitz studied institutionalized children and demonstrated that, due to lack of adequate nurturing, they become apathetic, withdrawn, and less interested in feeding, which in turn causes failure to thrive and, in extreme cases, death. Spitz called this syndrome anaclitic depression. Schizophrenia and autism have not been associated with emotional deprivation in infancy.

76. The answer is d. *(Kaplan and Sadock, p 206.)* Projection is recognized when a person perceives and reacts to an unacceptable inner impulse as if the impulse were coming from the external environment. In this case, the patient, likely with a huge amount of internal anger that she finds dangerous and unacceptable, projects this anger onto the therapist and reacts as if the therapist is angry at her. Distortion is the reshaping of external reality to suit one's inner needs. For example, a singer who is told at an audition that she needs a lot of work to make her voice stronger remembers the audition as notable for receiving only positive feedback. Blocking is the inhibition of thinking, temporarily and transiently. Isolation is the splitting or separating of an idea from the emotion that accompanies it (but has been repressed). Dissociation is the temporary but drastic modification of a person's sense of personal identity so that emotional distress can be avoided. Fugue states are one example of dissociation in action.

77. The answer is e. *(Kaplan and Sadock, p 28.)* The term *stranger anxiety* refers to manifestations of discomfort and distress on the part of the infant when he or she is approached by a stranger. Although it does not necessarily appear every time the child meets a stranger, and although some children seem to be more prone than others to such reactions, stranger anxiety is considered a normal, transient phenomenon. It manifests at about 8 months of age, when the child starts differentiating between familiar and unfamiliar adults.

78. The answer is b. (*Kaplan and Sadock, p 194.*) Primary process thinking is primitive, nonlogical, and timeless. Primary processes characterize the operational style of the id and are manifested in dreams. According to Freud's theory, condensation, displacement, and symbolic representation are forms of primary processes.

79. The answer is a. (*Kaplan and Sadock, p 201.*) In Freudian psychoanalytic theory, defense mechanisms represent the ego's attempts to mediate between the pressure of the instinctual drives, emerging from the id, and the restrictions imposed by societal rules through the superego. Freud classified defense mechanisms as narcissistic (or primitive, including denial, projection, and distortion), immature (acting out, introjection, passive-aggressive behavior, somatization, and several others), neurotic (displacement, externalization, intellectualization, rationalization, inhibition, reaction formation, and repression), and mature (sublimation, altruism, asceticism, anticipation, suppression, and humor). Primitive and immature defenses are the norm during childhood and infancy and persist in pathological states. Mature defenses are considered more adaptive than immature and neurotic defenses.

In displacement, an unacceptable impulse or emotion is shifted from one object to another. This permits the release of the impulse or emotion onto someone or something that is less dangerous. In this case, although the woman is angry at her boss, it is too dangerous to release this anger at him (she might be fired). She waits until she gets home and displaces this anger onto her husband. Projection is a defense mechanism in which the patient reacts to an inner unacceptable impulse as if it were outside the self.

80. The answer is c. (*Kaplan and Sadock, p 203.*) In reaction formation, an unacceptable unconscious impulse is transformed into its opposite. For example, a woman who is really angry at her neighbor begins to bring her flowers and cookies, while maintaining a "saccharine sweet" demeanor toward the neighbor. Rationalization refers to offering a rational explanation to justify actions or impulses that would otherwise be regarded as unacceptable.

81. The answer is b. (*Kaplan and Sadock, pp 202-204.*) Through sublimation, satisfaction of an objectionable impulse is obtained by using socially acceptable means. The writer in the question derives a vicarious satisfaction of his antisocial impulses through the criminal activities of the characters of his stories. Identification refers to the incorporation of another person's qualities into one's ego system. Introjection refers to the internalization of the qualities of an object. For example, through the introjection of a loved object, the painful awareness of separateness or the threat of loss may be avoided. Distortion refers to the gross reshaping of external reality to suit inner needs. Distortions include hallucinations and delusions.

82. The answer is d. (*Kaplan and Sadock, pp 202-204.*) Acting out means the avoidance of personally unacceptable feelings by behaving in a socially inappropriate manner that is often attention-seeking as well. Acting out implies the expression of an impulse through action to avoid experiencing the accompanying emotion related to that impulse at a conscious level. Intellectualization is the excessive use of intellectual processes to avoid affective expression or experience.

83. The answer is c. (*Kaplan and Sadock, pp 202-204.*) Intellectualization is the excessive use of intellectual processes to avoid affective expression or experience. In this case, the man avoids his guilty feelings through the meticulous explanation, over and over, of the events leading up to his car accident. Through sublimation, satisfaction of an objectionable impulse is obtained by using socially acceptable means. Repression refers to expelling or withholding from consciousness an idea or feeling. Acting out implies the expression of an impulse through action to avoid experiencing the accompanying effect at a conscious level. Rationalization is the process of offering rational explanations in an attempt to justify attitudes, beliefs, or behavior that may otherwise be unacceptable.

84. The answer is c. (*Kaplan and Sadock, p 581.*) Stress, such as this woman is experiencing secondary to her sudden illness and hospitalization, has long been known to cause a regression in cognitive and emotional functioning. The clue here is that her previous functioning, as described by her husband, was normal in both the cognitive and the emotional realms, making a previously undiagnosed personality disorder unlikely. Delirium would be accompanied by waxing and waning of consciousness, which is not described in this case. A mood disorder secondary to an organic cause is likewise unlikely, since the patient is not described as depressed or manic in behavior. Dissociation involves a person, under a sudden stressor that cannot be handled, switching to a distinctly different personality (and indeed, the patient might not remember a sense of "who she was" prior to the switch).

85. The answer is c. (*Kaplan and Sadock, pp 202-204.*) This woman is demonstrating undoing, a compulsive act that is performed in an attempt to negate or avoid the consequences of a fantasized action that is the result of an obsessional impulse. Although the fear is irrational, because the impulse is only a thought or fear and not an actual action, the compulsive nature of the act causes the person to perform it repeatedly regardless. Undoing is one of the three main psychological defense systems used in obsessive-compulsive disorder. The other two are isolation and reaction formation.

86. The answer is a. (*Kaplan and Sadock, p 140.*) This infant is displaying the protest phase of a separation, which occurs approximately 3 days after a young, well-attached child is separated from a parent. The protest phase is characterized by crying, calling, and searching for the parent. If the parent reappears shortly thereafter, before the child enters the despair phase of separation, the anger of the child is evidenced by his or her ambivalent response to the parent's return. This can be seen by the child refusing affection from the parent, turning his or her head away, and wanting to remain with the alternate caregiver. The despair phase, which follows the protest phase, is demonstrated by an air of hopelessness about the child, who even though still attached to the parent, may appear indifferent upon the parent's return. The fact that the child in this vignette actively refuses affection from his parent, and that there is no mention of the child appearing hopeless, makes it clear this child is still in the protest phase, and has not yet entered the despair phase. If the separation continues after a child has entered the despair phase, the child enters the detachment phase, when the bond with the parent has been irreparably severed.

87. The answer is e. (*Kaplan and Sadock, pp 133-137.*) The child is demonstrating that she recognizes object permanence, a level that is usually achieved at around 16 months. Prior to the achievement of this level, the child is unable to maintain a mental image of an object, so when it disappears from view, it, in effect, no longer exists. Once the child recognizes object permanence, he or she understands that objects can be hidden, thus making the game of hide-and-seek a rewarding one for a child of this age.

88. The answer is d. (*Kaplan and Sadock, pp 196-198.*) According to Freud's theory of psychosexual development, the child goes through six stages between birth and adolescence: oral, anal, phallic, oedipal, latency, and genital. In each stage, pleasure (not necessarily sexual) is derived from specific areas of the body. Each stage is associated with specific drives, conflicts, and defenses.

In the first 18 months of life, infants go through the oral stage, during which oral sensations (feeding, sucking, biting, etc) represent the main gratification. According to Freud, excessive gratification or deprivation during this stage can cause an "oral fixation." Individuals with an oral character are dependent and require that others fulfill their needs. In the anal stage, between 18 and 36 months of age, the child is much more independent and active than during the previous stage. Erotic stimulation of the anal mucosa through the excretion or retention of feces is the main source of pleasure. Battles over toilet training are common in the attempts to achieve autonomy from the parents. If toilet training is too harsh or inconsistent, "anal traits" may persist as personality traits later in life. Stubbornness, obstinacy, and frugality are common traits of the "anal individual," usually seen in obsessive-compulsive personalities. The phallic stage, which starts at age 3, is characterized by a concentration of erotic pleasure in the penis and the clitoris areas. During the phallic stage, the child starts looking outside himself or herself for an erotic object, thus heralding the advent of the oedipal stage. Freud theorized that between the ages of 3 and 5, the male child, like Oedipus in Greek mythology, falls in love with the mother and perceives the father as a murderous rival. Resolution of the oedipal stage leads to the boy's identification with the father and the abandonment of the erotic wishes for the mother, which are later transferred to other women. During the oedipal stage, girls experience an equivalent attraction for their fathers and perceive their mothers as rivals. How girls resolve their oedipal conflicts and come to identify with their mothers is less clearly explained. During latency, between 5 and 11 to 13 years of age, the sexual drive is relatively quiescent and the child becomes focused on learning new skills and social interactions with peers. The genital stage begins with puberty and ends with young adulthood and is characterized by a reintensification of sexual drives. The key developmental tasks associated with this stage are mastery over instinctual drives, separation from parents, and the establishment of a genital sexuality with an appropriate partner.

89. The answer is d. (*Kaplan and Sadock, pp 193-194.*) The topographic model of the mind divides the mind into three regions: the conscious (that part of the mind in which perceptions coming from the outside world or from within the body or mind are brought into awareness), the preconscious (those mental events, processes, and contents capable of being brought into conscious awareness by the act of focusing attention), and the unconscious (mental contents and processes kept from conscious awareness through the force of censorship or repression). Parapraxes are unwitting slips of the tongue that reveal the unconscious at work. Infantile sexuality is a Freudian developmental theory of childhood sexuality that delineates the vicissitudes of erotic activity from birth through puberty. The structural theory of the mind describes the three psychic apparatuses—the ego, the id, and the superego—all distinguished by their different functions. Primary process refers to thinking that is dereistic, illogical, or magical; it is normally found in dreams and abnormally in psychosis.

90. The answer is b. *(Kaplan and Sadock, p 32.)* Going to school is the major developmental event of middle childhood, which is typically described as the period of time between ages 6 and 12. The onset of puberty and the development of an overt interest in the opposite sex typically occur later, in adolescence (ages 12 to15). The consolidation of personality and a growing concern with cultural values and ideologies occur in late adolescence, typically defined as 17 to 20 years of age.

Human Behavior: Biologic and Related Sciences

Questions

91. A 24-year-old man is diagnosed with schizophrenia. He enters a research study looking at dopamine activity in the central nervous system. Which of the following substances will undoubtedly be examined in the young man's cerebrospinal fluid, blood, or urine?

a. Monoamine oxidase
b. Tyrosine
c. Homovanillic acid
d. Tyrosine hydroxylase
e. DOPA (3,4-dihydroxyphenylalanine)

92. A young man is often the object of his friends' jokes because he drops to the floor whenever he is having a good laugh. From which of the following is this man most likely suffering?

a. Cataplexy
b. Narcolepsy
c. Hysteria
d. Drop seizures
e. Histrionic personality

93. A 78-year-old man is brought to the physician by his wife because he is becoming increasingly confused. He has been found wandering along the streets unable to find his way home, and has left items in unusual places, like putting his sunglasses in the freezer. On mental status examination the physician would like to test for diffuse cortical degeneration. Which of the following would most likely demonstrate this problem if it is present?

a. Ask the patient about presence of hallucinations.
b. Ask the patient to pick up a piece of paper in his left hand, fold it in half, and place it back on the table.
c. Ask the patient to spell the word 'WORLD' backward.
d. Ask the patient to copy a figure with multiple intersecting lines.
e. Ask the patient to tell the physician what year he and his wife were married.

94. An 18-year-old man is admitted to the psychiatric unit after his parents find him in his room muttering to himself and convinced that people are going to hurt him. During his stay in the hospital, the patient is frequently found standing in the center of his room with both arms over his head, immobile. The patient can maintain this position for hours at a time. Which of the following best describes this patient's posturing?

a. Negativism
b. Automatism
c. Stereotypy
d. Waxy flexibility
e. Catalepsy

95. A 25-year-old woman is seen by a psychiatrist because her family says that she is "hyperintense" about everything. On interview the patient denies mood swings, though does note that she is "emotionally intense." She denies hallucinations, delusions, suicidal or homicidal ideation. She is noted to be very "perseverative" in her interaction with the psychiatrist, pursuing even small points of discussion further and further so that very little ground can be covered during the interview. She denies having any medical problems, though does state that a neurologist told her that her EEG was "abnormal." However, she denies ever having any seizures during which she lost consciousness. Which of the following might be affecting this patient?

a. Temporal lobe epilepsy
b. Kluver-Bucy syndrome
c. Damage to the amygdale
d. Damage to the left hemisphere
e. Diffuse cortical atrophy

96. Benzodiazepines, barbiturates, and many anticonvulsants exert their influence through which of the following types of receptors?

a. Muscarinic
b. Dopaminergic
c. Glutamic
d. Adrenergic
e. γ-Aminobutyric acid (GABA)–ergic

97. A 32-year-old man is brought to the emergency room unresponsive. Shortly after arriving at the emergency room, he stops breathing. The patient's friends state that the patient has a long history of depression and anxiety and is taking fluoxetine. They state that just prior to the man becoming unresponsive, he was at a party and was drinking alcohol, though they did not think that he drank more than two or three drinks. The patient's toxicology screen reveals, in addition to the substances listed above, the presence of cocaine, benzodiazepines, and marijuana. What is the most likely reason that this patient stopped breathing?

a. The patient used cocaine and benzodiazepines.
b. The patient used marijuana and alcohol.
c. The patient used fluoxetine and benzodiazepines.
d. The patient used fluoxetine and alcohol.
e. The patient used benzodiazepines and alcohol.

98. The observation that levodopa (a drug used to treat Parkinson disease) can cause mania and psychosis in some patients supports which neurochemical theory of psychiatric behavior?

a. Norepinephrine
b. Dopamine
c. Glycine
d. Serotonin
e. Glutamine

99. A 42-year-old woman is involved in a motorcycle accident, in which she sustains permanent damage to her inferolateral temporal lobes. On subsequent mental status examination, which elements of this patient's memory will be found to be impaired?

a. Episodic memory
b. Semantic memory
c. Procedural memory
d. Immediate memory
e. Working memory

100. A 46-year-old man is being monitored in a sleep study laboratory. After he has been asleep for 90 minutes, his EEG shows low-voltage, random fast activity with sawtooth waves. When awakened during this period, the patient reports that he was dreaming. Which of the following sleep stages was this patient in when awakened?

a. Alpha waves
b. Theta waves
c. Sleep spindles
d. Delta waves
e. Rapid eye movement (REM)

101. A 56-year-old man is admitted to the hospital after a stroke. The stroke is localized to the border of the somatosensory and association areas in the posterior parietal lobe. Which of the following symptoms would be displayed upon neurological testing?

a. Loss of proprioception
b. Loss of vibratory sensation
c. Loss of the ability to recognize items based on touch
d. Loss of pressure sensation
e. Loss of pain sensation

102. After being struck on the head by a four-by-four piece of wood, a previously serious and dependable construction worker starts making inappropriate sexual remarks to his coworkers, is easily distracted, and loses his temper over minor provocations. What part of his brain has most likely been damaged?

a. Occipital lobe
b. Temporal lobe
c. Limbic system
d. Basal ganglion
e. Frontal lobe

Questions 103 to 111

Match each of the following receptor subtypes with the appropriate clinical scenario which is affected by that receptor. Each lettered option may be used once, more than once, or not at all.

a. Serotonin receptor, Subtype 5-HT$_{1A}$
b. Serotonin receptor, Subtype 5-HT$_{1D}$
c. Serotonin receptor, Subtype 5-HT$_6$
d. Serotonin receptor, Subtype 5-HT$_7$
e. Histamine, Subtype H$_1$
f. Dopamine, Subtype D$_2$
g. Dopamine, Subtype D$_4$
h. Adrenergic transmitter, Subtype $\alpha_{1A,B,D}$
i. Adrenergic transmitter, Subtype β_2
j. Cholinergic transmitter, Subtype M$_4$

103. A 25-year-old woman comes to the neurologist for treatment of her migraine headaches. She is prescribed sumatriptan.

104. A 19-year-old man is admitted to the psychiatry unit after he is brought to the hospital by police. On admission, he admitted to hearing voices and seeing "the devil." His parents say that he has begun acting strangely and more withdrawn over the past 7 months. He is started on risperidone.

105. A 39-year-old shift worker comes to his primary care doctor because he is having trouble adjusting to his new night shift schedule.

106. A 42-year-old man comes to the physician for a 3-month history of frequent headaches and fatigue. He is found to have a blood pressure of 185/98 mm/Hg and is started on an antihypertensive medication.

107. A 36-year-old woman comes to the psychiatrist for a 3-month history of increasing anxiety, ever since her husband was laid off from work. She states that she has always been a "worrier" but that now her anxiety is just not manageable on her own. She is started on Buspirone.

108. A 20-year-old woman is started on an inhaler medication to help with her asthma.

109. A 52-year-old man is newly diagnosed with Parkinson disease. He is particularly bothered by the involuntary resting tremor. He is started on benztropine and the symptoms improve.

110. A 38-year-old chronic schizophrenic comes to the emergency department because he is out of his medications. He tells the emergency room doctor that his medication, haloperidol, works really well for his auditory hallucinations, but it also gives him a "twisted neck" on occasion.

111. A 25-year-old woman comes to her physician with complaints of sedation and weight gain since she started using diphenhydramine for her seasonal allergies.

112. A young girl who was underweight and hypotonic in infancy is obsessed with food, eats compulsively, and at age 4, is already grossly overweight. She is argumentative, oppositional, and rigid. She has a narrow face, almond-shaped eyes, and a small mouth. Which of the following is the most likely diagnosis?

a. Down syndrome
b. Fragile X syndrome
c. Fetal alcohol syndrome
d. Hypothyroidism
e. Prader-Willi syndrome

Questions 113 to 123

Match the following terms with the deficits which they describe. Each lettered option may be used once, more than once, or not at all.

a. Prosopagnosia
b. Apperceptive visual agnosia
c. Associative visual agnosia
d. Color agnosia
e. Color anomia
f. Central achromatopsia
g. Anton syndrome
h. Balint syndrome
i. Oculomotor apraxia
j. Simultanagnosia
k. Gerstmann syndrome

113. Complete inability to perceive color.

114. Inability to integrate a visual scene to perceive it as a whole.

115. Agraphia, acalculia, right-left disorientation, and finger angosia.

116. Inability to identify and draw items using visual cues, with preservation of other sensory modalities.

117. Inability to name a color despite the ability to point at it.

118. Inability to direct gaze rapidly.

119. Inability to recognize faces.

120. Inability to recognize a color despite being able to match it.

121. Triad of the inability to direct optically guided movements, the inability to direct gaze rapidly, and the inability to integrate a visual scene to perceive it as a whole.

122. The failure to acknowledge blindness.

123. Inability to name or use objects despite the ability to draw them.

124. A 36-year-old moderately retarded man with a long head, large ears, and hyperextensible joints is very shy and starts rocking and flapping his hands when he is upset. Which of the following disorders produces this symptom constellation?

a. Down syndrome
b. Hurler syndrome
c. Williams syndrome
d. Fragile X syndrome
e. Rett disorder

125. Monoamine oxidase inhibitors (MAOIs) exert their influence primarily by which of the following mechanisms?

a. Increasing GABA production
b. Blocking inactivation of biogenic amines
c. Decreasing norepinephrine
d. Decreasing serotonin
e. Increasing endorphin production

126. A 36-year-old woman is being evaluated in the sleep laboratory. She is noted to have a decreased latency of REM. Which of the following disorders is this woman most likely to be suffering from?

a. Schizophrenia
b. Major depression
c. Panic disorder
d. Obsessive-compulsive disorder
e. Posttraumatic stress disorder (PTSD)

127. A 17-year-old boy is brought to the emergency room by his friends after he "took a few pills" at a party and developed physical symptoms, including his neck twisting to one side, his eyes rolling upward, and his tongue hanging out of his mouth. The patient responds immediately to 50 mg of diphenhydramine intramuscularly with the resolution of all physical symptoms. Which of the following substances is most likely to have caused the symptoms?

a. Methamphetamine
b. Meperidine
c. Alprazolam
d. Methylphenidate
e. Haloperidol

128. A 52-year-old housewife has gained weight, although she does not note an increased appetite. She states she feels tired all the time and does not care about hobbies that she enjoyed previously. On physical examination, her skin appears dry and her hair is brittle. She appears depressed although she denies suicidal ideation. Which of the following laboratory findings is she likely to display?

a. Elevated adrenocorticotropic hormone (ACTH)
b. Low cortisol level
c. Elevated thyroid-stimulating hormone (TSH)
d. Low calcium level
e. Elevated follicle-stimulating hormone (FSH)

129. A 32-year-old woman is brought to the emergency room when she complains of chest pain. She is noted to be hypervigilant and anxious, with a pulse of 120 beats/minute and BP of 140/97 mm/Hg. Her temperature is not elevated. She has widely dilated pupils. Her toxicology screen is positive. Which of the following drugs is she most likely to have used?

a. Cocaine
b. Ritalin
c. Heroin
d. Phencyclidine (PCP)
e. Lysergic acid diethylamide (LSD)

130. A 28-year-old woman comes to her psychiatrist for a renewal of her prescription for haloperidol. She has been on this drug for 6 months after she was hospitalized for a psychotic episode. She complains to the psychiatrist about a white milky discharge from both of her breasts. What is the mechanism of action which is causing this medication-induced effect?

a. The patient has had the D_2 receptors at the end of the nigrostriatal tract blocked by the antipsychotic drug.
b. The patient has had the amount of serotonin increased in the synaptic cleft of the neurons in the caudate nucleus.
c. The haloperidol has acted upon peptide receptors, which project to practically every brain region.
d. Homovanillic acid levels have increased in the cerebrospinal fluid.
e. The blockade of dopamine receptors in the tuberoinfundibular tract eliminated the inhibitory effect of dopamine on prolactin release.

131. A 42-year-old woman comes to the psychiatrist with complaints of short-term memory loss. She has lost her way home several times in past weeks. Mini Mental Status Exam scores 18 of 30 points. An MRI shows the loss of brain volume. The patient's mother died of the same disease at age 46. Which of the following genes in this patient (and her mother) are likely to show a mutation on chromosome 14?

a. *Presinilin 1*
b. *Presinilin 2*
c. *β-Amyloid precursor protein (APP)*
d. *Apolipoprotein E (Apo E)*
e. *Human lymphocyte antigen (HLA)*

132. A 24-year-old woman comes to the emergency room because she "can't stand the addiction to cocaine anymore." She tells the physician that she has been using cocaine in increasing amounts for the past 2 years, and now her use is totally out of control. Which of the following systems is involved in this drug's capacity for such a high addiction potential in human beings?

a. Serotonergic
b. GABA-ergic
c. Dopaminergic
d. Noradrenergic
e. Biogenic amine system

133. A 50-year-old man notes that several times per week he has a hallucination of the smell of burning rubber. He is diagnosed with partial complex seizures. Which of the following regions is most likely to show a discharging focus on EEG?

a. Parietal lobe
b. Temporal lobe
c. Frontal lobe
d. Thalamus
e. Occipital lobe

134. Which of the following findings is associated with non-REM (NREM) sleep?

a. Penile tumescence
b. Apnea
c. Narcolepsy
d. Dreaming
e. Night terrors

135. A 48-year-old man is being treated for a major depression. He complains of depressed mood, anergia, anhedonia, and suicidal ideation with a plan. Which of the following neurochemicals is likely to be abnormal in this patient's CSF?

a. 5-Hydroxyindoleacetic acid (5-HIAA)
b. GABA
c. Dopamine
d. Acetylcholine
e. Substance P

136. A 34-year-old man comes to see a psychiatrist because he has been fired for constantly being late to his job. The man states that he feels as if he is in danger of contamination from germs and as a result, he must take showers continuously, often for as many as 8 hours/day. Which of the following transmitters is thought to be involved in this disorder?

a. Dopamine
b. Norepinephrine
c. Acetylcholine
d. Histamine
e. Serotonin

137. A 71-year-old man has been treated by a neurologist for Parkinson disease for the past 2 years. One week after his last visit, he called his neurologist, reporting that he suddenly began seeing little people walking all over his furniture. The patient had never previously reported symptoms as described. Which of the following is the most appropriate next step in the management of this patient?

a. Reduce the L-dopa
b. Increase the L-dopa
c. Add haloperidol
d. Add Sinemet
e. Call a psychiatrist for consultation

138. A 76-year-old man is diagnosed with dementia of the Alzheimer type. Which of the following chemicals has been most commonly associated with this disease?

a. Peptide neurotransmitter
b. Epinephrine
c. Dopamine
d. Acetylcholine
e. Serotonin

Questions 139 to 141

Match the correct substance with the questions below. Each lettered option may be used once, more than once, or not at all.

a. Neuropeptide Y
b. GABA
c. Norepinephrine
d. Somatostatin
e. Substance P
f. Glutamate
g. Acetylcholine
h. Serotonin

139. Which of these substances is most associated with the classic antidepressant drugs, as well as venlafaxine, mirtazapine, and bupropion?

140. Which of these substances is most prominently associated with the mediation of the perception of pain?

141. Which of these substances has been shown to stimulate the appetite?

Questions 142 and 143

A 47-year-old man is referred to a physician for evaluation of new-onset aphasia. Match each of the following symptom presentations with the corresponding type of aphasia. Each lettered option may be used once, more than once, or not at all.

a. Broca
b. Wernicke
c. Conduction
d. Global
e. Anomic

142. Fluent spontaneous speech, poor auditory comprehension, poor repetition, poor naming.

143. Nonfluent spontaneous speech, good auditory comprehension, poor repetition, poor naming.

144. Which of the following sites is thought to be significant for formation and storage of immediate and recent memories?

a. Hypothalamus
b. Nucleus basalis of Meynert
c. Mesolimbic circuit
d. Hippocampus
e. Amygdala

145. A 54-year-old man is a chronic alcoholic. He has been diagnosed with Korsakoff syndrome (a severe inability to form new memories and a variable inability to recall remote memories). Where in the brain is the damage causing this memory loss likely located?

a. Angular gyrus
b. Mammillary bodies
c. Hypothalamus
d. Globus pallidus
e. Arcuate fasciculus

146. A 35-year-old man presents to his physician with a slowly developing difficulty of movement and thinking. The patient tells the physician that his father had similar problems. His wife notes that the patient appears depressed and apathetic. On examination, the patient has involuntary choreiform movements of his face, hands, and shoulders. Which of the following areas of the brain is likely to show atrophy with this disease?

a. Caudate nucleus
b. Frontal lobe(s)
c. White matter
d. Cerebellum
e. Pituitary

147. A 58-year-old man has a brain lesion that causes him to feel euphoric, laugh uncontrollably, and joke and make puns. Where is this brain lesion most likely located?

a. Fornix
b. Right prefrontal cortex
c. Hippocampus
d. Left orbitofrontal cortex
e. Amygdala

148. A 28-year-old man with a 6-month history of symptoms is noted to have disinhibition, lability, and euphoria. He is also noted to have a lack of remorse. Which area of the man's brain is likely to be dysfunctional?

a. Orbitofrontal region of frontal lobe
b. Dorsolateral region of frontal lobe
c. Medial region of frontal lobe
d. Limbic system
e. Parietal lobe

149. A 44-year-old man has had a traumatic injury to his brain. Since the accident, he has appeared inattentive and undermotivated. He tends to linger on trivial thoughts and echoes the examiner's questions. Which area of the man's brain is likely to have been traumatized?

a. Orbitofrontal region of frontal lobe
b. Dorsolateral region of frontal lobe
c. Medial region of frontal lobe
d. Limbic system
e. Parietal lobe

150. A 48-year-old man with Huntington disease experiences irregular, involuntary spasmodic movements of his limbs and facial muscles, as well as psychosis. In a postmortem autopsy, which structure in his brain will likely be markedly shrunken?

a. Cerebellum
b. Striatum
c. Putamen
d. Substantia nigra
e. Caudate nucleus

Questions 151 to 156

Match the correct deficiency or excess with the symptom constellations below. Each lettered option may be used once, more than once, or not at all.

a. Vitamin A excess
b. Vitamin B_{12} deficiency
c. Folate deficiency
d. Thiamine deficiency
e. Vitamin D excess
f. Vitamin E excess

151. A 22-year-old woman with celiac disease delivers a full-term infant with a neural tube defect. The woman complains of headaches, a sore tongue, irritability, and heart palpitations.

152. A 42-year-old body builder complains of weakness, nausea, vomiting, headaches, and constipation. He also has polyuria and polydipsia. He is found to have excessive calcification of bone and soft tissue, as well as kidney stones.

153. A 51-year-old homeless man is found wandering in the middle of the street and is brought to the emergency room. On mental status examination, he is found to confabulate, admits to auditory hallucinations, and has a severe loss of memory. On examination, he is found to be ataxic.

154. A 26-year-old woman presents with dry and itchy skin, hair loss, headaches, visual changes, bone and muscle pain, fatigue, irritability, and anemia. Her conjunctivae have a yellow tone. She states that she has been taking a variety of oral supplements in order to "stay healthy."

155. A 62-year-old man is admitted to the hospital after a hemorrhagic stroke. He states that prior to the stroke, he noted weakness, fatigue, nausea, and diarrhea. He also noted that he was bruising extremely easily. He stated that he had been taking high doses of supplements for a number of years to "protect my heart."

156. A 39-year-old strict vegan presents with irritability, problems with concentration, and a depressed mood with suicidal ideation. On examination she is found to have an abnormal neurological examination, with decreased tendon reflexes, and impairments in the perception of deep touch, pressure, and vibration. She has an anemia on laboratory evaluation as well.

Questions 157 to 163

Match the following serotonin receptor sites, which when activated, produce the listed side effects. Each lettered option may be used once, more than once, or not at all.

a. Basal ganglia
b. Brain stem (area postrema)
c. Limbic system
d. Brain stem (sleep center)
e. Spinal cord pathway
f. Intestines
g. Cranial blood vessels

157. Initial increase in anxiety after being started on the drug

158. Gastrointestinal upset and diarrhea

159. Headache

160. Akathisia and agitation

161. Nausea and vomiting

162. Insomnia or somnolence

163. Sexual dysfunction

Questions 164 to 168

Match the following diagnoses with their characteristic findings on MRI. Each lettered option may be used once, more than once, or not at all.

a. Periventricular patches of increased signal intensity
b. Atrophy of caudate nucleus
c. Enhancement of the meninges at the base of the brain
d. Dilatation of the ventricles
e. Patches of increased signal in the white matter (not periventricular only)

164. A 29-year-old man is diagnosed with chronic neurosyphilis.

165. A 40-year-old woman presents to the physician with symptoms of dementia and a gait disorder.

166. A 36-year-old man presents with weakness in his right arm and visual difficulties in his right eye.

167. A 40-year-old man presents with a movement disorder. He notes that this condition runs in his family.

168. A 72-year-old woman is brought to the physician by her husband, who notes that she is increasingly unable to care for herself.

Questions 169 to 172

Match the following EEG wave forms with their characteristic properties. Each lettered option may be used once, more than once, or not at all.
a. Alpha
b. Beta
c. Delta
d. Theta

169. Dominant brain wave frequency (8 to 13 Hz) of the normal, eyes-closed, awake EEG.

170. Frequency is faster than 13 Hz; not uncommon in normal adult waking EEGs, particularly over the frontal-central regions.

171. Prominently featured in deeper stages of sleep. Frequency of less than 3.5 Hz.

172. Waves with a frequency of 4.0 to 7.5 Hz. Prominent feature of the drowsy and sleep tracing.

Human Behavior: Biologic and Related Sciences

Answers

91. The answer is c. *(Kaplan and Sadock, p 100.)* Homovanillic acid is the primary metabolite of dopamine. Dopamine activity in the CNS is often assessed in research studies by looking for this metabolite in the cerebrospinal fluid, blood, or urine.

92. The answer is a. *(Kaplan and Sadock, p 760.)* Cataplexy refers to a sudden loss of muscle tone (ranging in severity from weakness in the knee to a total loss of tone) triggered by strong emotions, which takes place during full wakefulness. Cataplexy is thought to be because of an abnormal intrusion of REM sleep phenomena in periods of wakefulness. It is usually treated with medications that reduce REM sleep, such as antidepressants. Cataplexy may be a symptom of narcolepsy, another dyssomnia characterized by the irresistible urge to fall asleep regardless of the situation.

93. The answer is b. *(Kaplan and Sadock, p 78.)* Ideational apraxia is the inability to put a sequence of skilled acts together in a row, though the individual may be able to perform each component of the sequence without error. The motor sequence representation of these acts may involve the left parietal cortex, as well as the sequencing and executive functions of the prefrontal cortex. This apraxia is a typical finding in those with cortical degeneration from Alzheimer disease.

94. The answer is e. *(Kaplan and Sadock, pp 273-283.)* Catalepsy refers to an immobile position that is constantly maintained, as is the case with this patient. Negativism is a resistance to any and all attempts to have the patient move or allow himself or herself to be moved—even when there is no obvious motive for such resistance. An automatism is the automatic performance of an act or acts, and it is thought that the act or acts have some kind of unconscious symbolic meaning. Stereotypy is a repetitive and fixed pattern of behavior or speech. Waxy flexibility (cerea flexibilitas) is the condition in which a person can literally be molded (as one would mold wax) into any position the examiner chooses, and this position is then maintained.

95. The answer is a. (*Kaplan and Sadock, pp 88-89.*) This patient is likely suffering from temporal lobe epilepsy, and she demonstrates a TLE personality, characterized by hyposexuality, emotional intensity, and viscosity, a peculiar perseverative approach to interactions with others. Kluver-Bucy patients might exhibit an almost opposite personality, with hypersexuality, placidity, constantly shifting attention, and a tendency to put everything in the patient's mouth. Damage to the amygdala might render patients unable to recognize fear or anger in others, though they remain able to recognize happiness and sadness. Damage to the left hemisphere produces intellectual dysfunction, and diffuse cortical atrophy produces symptoms consistent with a picture of Alzheimer patient.

96. The answer is e. (*Kaplan and Sadock, pp 108-109.*) GABA receptors represent the most important inhibitory system in the central nervous system (CNS) and are found in almost every area of the brain. Benzodiazepines, barbiturates, and many anticonvulsants act through activation of the GABA receptors. This explains the cross-tolerance that occurs between these substances.

97. The answer is e. (*Kaplan and Sadock, p 395.*) While benzodiazepines are generally recognized to be extremely safe medications, when taken in an overdose in combination with alcohol they can be particularly dangerous. Alcohol has an additive effect to the CNS and respiratory depressant effects of benzodiazepines, because it increases the binding affinity of benzodiazepines to the benzodiazepine-binding site.

98. The answer is b. (*Kaplan and Sadock, pp 102-103.*) Levodopa is a chemical relative of dopamine. The fact that a dopamine-related compound can cause psychotic symptoms in some patients supports the dopamine hypothesis of schizophrenia, which is the leading neurochemical hypothesis for this disease.

99. The answer is b. (*Kaplan and Sadock, p 87.*) There are three major categories of memory: episodic, semantic, and procedural. In addition, there are three major periods of memory: immediate (functioning over a period of seconds), recent (minutes to days), and remote (months to years). All the types and periods of memory have distinct anatomical correlates. Episodic memory is sited in the medial temporal lobes, the anterior thalamic nucleus, mamillary body, fornix, and prefrontal cortex. Semantic memory is located in the inferolateral temporal lobes and is responsible for allowing patients to correctly answer such questions as the color of a certain breed of dog, or how an orange and an apple are different. Procedural memory, as the name implies, allows one to remember how to drive a car or remember the phone number of a friend. Such memory is located in the basal ganglia, cerebellum, and supplementary motor area. Working memory is the ability to store information for several seconds while other cognitive activities work on the information.

100. The answer is e. *(Kaplan and Sadock, pp 751-752.)* Dreaming is the main characteristic of REM sleep. The EEG shows characteristic low-voltage waves that are random, fast, and sawtoothed. Active eye movements are attributed to the individual's "watching" his or her dreams. A lack of muscle tone during REM sleep prevents the individual from acting out his or her dreams. REM sleep is also characterized by increased heart rate and blood pressure and penile or clitoral nocturnal erections.

101. The answer is c. *(Kaplan and Sadock, pp 71-72).* Tactile agnosia (astereognosis) is defined as the inability to recognize objects based on touch. Damage to the border of the somatosensory and association areas in the posterior parietal lobe appear to cause a failure of the highest level of feature extraction (that of the ability to recognize objects by touch) while preserving the more basic features of the somatosensory pathway (ie, light touch, pressure, pain, vibration, temperature, and position sense).

102. The answer is e. *(Kaplan and Sadock, pp 88-89.)* The frontal lobes are associated with the regulation of emotions, the manifestation of behavioral traits usually connected to the personality of an individual, and executive functions (the ability to make appropriate judgments and decisions and to form concepts). They also contain the inhibitory systems for behaviors such as bladder and bowel release. Damage of the frontal lobes causes impairment of these functions but it is not, strictly speaking, a form of dementia, because memory, language, calculation ability, praxis, and IQ are often preserved. Personality changes, disinhibited behavior, and poor judgment are usually seen with lesions of the dorsolateral regions of the frontal lobes. Lesions of the mesial region, which is involved in the regulation of the initiation of movements and emotional responses, cause slowing of motor functions, speech, and emotional reactions. In the most severe cases, patients are mute and akinetic. Lesions of the orbitofrontal area are accompanied by abnormal social behaviors, an excessively good opinion of oneself, jocularity, sexual disinhibition, and lack of concern for others. The occipital lobe is the visual processing center, containing most of the visual cortex. The temporal lobe contains the auditory cortex, and is also involved in the formation of long-term memories. The limbic system is a complicated, multi-functional area of the brain responsible for the control of emotions, olfaction, long-term memory, and behavior. The basal ganglion are also multi-functional, involved in the control of emotions, procedural movements of routine behaviors, and voluntary movements.

103 to 111. The answers are 103-b, 104-c or g, 105-d, 106-h, 107-a, 108-i, 109-j, 110-f, 111-e *(Kaplan and Sadock, p 99.)* The serotonin receptor, Subtype 5-HT_{1D} is the target of the anti-migraine drug sumatriptan. The serotonin receptor, Subtype 5-H_{T6} is the target of the atypical antipsychotics, such as risperidone. In addition, the dopamine receptor D_4 is also the target of the atypical antipsychotics, so the answer to question 104 is correctly stated as both c and g. Serotonin receptor 5-HT_7 is implicated in the regulation of circadian rhythms. Antihypertensives work at the adrenergic transmitter, Subtype $\alpha_{1A,B,D}$. The serotonin receptor, Subtype 5-HT_{1A} has anxiolytic properties. The adrenergic transmitter, Subtype β_2, is responsible for the regulation of bronchial muscle contraction. The cholinergic transmitter, Subtype M_4, is the target of antiparkinsonism anticholinergic drugs. The dopamine, Subtype D_2 receptor is the target of therapeutic and extrapyramidal effects of dopamine receptor antagonists like haloperidol, which are "typical antipsychotics." Antagonists to the histamine, Subtype H_1 receptor, such as diphenhydramine, produce sedation and weight gain.

112. The answer is e. *(Kaplan and Sadock, p 1142.)* Prader-Willi syndrome is a genetic disorder caused by a defect of the long arm of chromosome 15. Characteristically, children are underweight in infancy. In early childhood, owing to a hypothalamic dysfunction, they start eating voraciously and quickly become grossly overweight. Individuals with this syndrome have characteristic facial features and present with a variety of neurologic and neuropsychiatric symptoms including autonomic dysregulation, muscle weakness, hypotonia, mild to moderate mental retardation, temper tantrums, violent outbursts, perseveration, skin picking, and a tendency to be argumentative, oppositional, and rigid.

113-123. The answers are 113-f, 114-j, 115-k, 116-b, 117-e, 118-i, 119-a, 120-d, 121-h, 122-g, 123-c *(Kaplan and Sadock, p 75.)* Central achromatopsia is a complete inability to perceive color. Simultanagnosia is the inability to integrate a visual scene to perceive it as a whole. Gerstmann syndrome includes agraphia, calculation difficulties (acalculia), right-left disorientation, and finger agnosia. It is thought to be related to lesions of the parietal lobe, dominant hemisphere. Apperceptive visual agnosia is the inability to identify and draw items using visual cues, though other sensory modalities are preserved. Color anomia is the inability to name a color despite being able to point to it. Oculomotor apraxia is the inability to direct gaze rapidly. Prosopagnosia is the inability to recognize faces in the presence of preserved recognition of other objects. It is thought to result from the disconnect of the left inferior temporal cortices (ITC) from the visual association area in the left parietal lobe. Color agnosia is the inability to recognize a color despite being able to match it. Balint syndrome, seen in bilateral parieto-occipital lesions, is a triad of optic ataxia (inability to direct optically guided movements), oculomotor apraxia, and simultanagnosia. Anton syndrome is a failure to acknowledge blindness, seen with bilateral occipital lobe lesions. Associative visual agnosia is the inability to name or use objects despite the ability to draw them and is caused by bilateral medial occipitotemporal lesions.

124. The answer is d. *(Kaplan and Sadock, pp 1141-1145.)* Fragile X syndrome is the most common form of inherited mental retardation, with a prevalence of 1 in 1200 in males and 1 in 2500 in females. Its manifestations are because of the inactivation of the fragile X mental retardation gene. Affected individuals have characteristic physical features including long face, large ears, and large hands. Adult males also have enlarged testicles owing to elevated gonadotropin levels. Affected individuals and female carriers have higher rates of obsessive-compulsive disorder (OCD), attention deficit hyperactivity disorder (ADHD), dysthymia, anxiety, and antisocial personality disorder. Individuals with fragile X syndrome also display many behaviors reminiscent of autism. They are shy and socially awkward, they avoid eye contact, and as autistic individuals, they engage in self-stimulatory, peculiar, and self-injurious behaviors. Down syndrome is the most common genetic mental retardation syndrome, occurring in 1 in 660 live births, but in the majority of cases (94%) it is caused by a de novo trisomy of chromosome 21 and, as such, it is not inherited. Hurler syndrome is one of the mucopolysaccharidoses. In its most severe form, this rare syndrome presents with multisystemic deterioration secondary to the accumulation of mucopolysaccharides. Hurler syndrome starts during the first year of life and causes death before age 10. Rett syndrome, a pervasive developmental disorder, is characterized by a devastating progressive deterioration of cognitive, social, and motor functions that starts between the ages of 5 months and 18 months, after an initial period of normal development. Williams syndrome is a rare form of genetic mental retardation caused by a deletion of part of chromosome 23.

125. The answer is b. *(Kaplan and Sadock, pp 1066-1070.)* Monoamine oxidases inactivate biogenic amines such as norepinephrine, serotonin, dopamine, and tyramine through oxidative deamination. The MAOIs block this inactivation, thereby increasing the availability of these neurotransmitters for synaptic release.

126. The answer is b. *(Kaplan and Sadock, p 531.)* A decreased latency of REM sleep is seen in major depression. Depression is the psychiatric disorder that has been most associated with disruptions in biological rhythms. Besides the decreased latency of REM sleep, early morning awakening and other neuroendocrine perturbations are often found with major depression.

127. The answer is e. *(Kaplan and Sadock, pp 992-993.)* The boy in the question experienced an acute dystonic reaction, an adverse effect of neuroleptic medications secondary to blockage of dopamine receptors in the nigrostriatal system. Dystonic reactions are sustained spasmodic contractions of the muscles of the neck, trunk, tongue, face, and extraocular muscles. They can be quite painful and frightening. They usually occur within hours to 3 days after the beginning of the treatment and are more frequent in males and young people. They are also usually associated with high-potency neuroleptics. Occasionally, dystonic reactions are seen in young people who have ingested a neuroleptic medication, mistaking it for a drug of abuse. Administration of anticholinergic drugs provides rapid treatment of acute dystonia.

128. The answer is c. *(Kaplan and Sadock, pp 820-821.)* The symptoms experienced by the woman in the question are prototypical for hypothyroidism, though the patient might be suffering from a major depression instead (since there are no blood tests to rule in or out a major depression, one would rule in or out likely medical conditions first before making that diagnosis in this case). Depressive symptoms are commonly associated with hypothyroidism. Hypocalcemia and hypercortisolemia (associated with an elevated ACTH in Cushing syndrome) are also associated with depression but present with different symptoms.

129. The answer is a. (*Kaplan and Sadock, p 914.*) Cocaine inhibits the normal reuptake of norepinephrine and dopamine, causing an increased concentration of these neurotransmitters in the synaptic cleft. This mechanism is responsible for the euphoria and sense of well-being that follow cocaine use, but it also causes excessive sympathetic activation and diffuse vasoconstriction. High blood pressure, mydriasis, cardiac arrhythmias, coronary artery spasms, and myocardial infarcts are all seen with cocaine intoxication. Other toxic effects of cocaine include headaches, ischemic cerebral and spinal infarcts, subarachnoid hemorrhages, and seizures. Intoxication with methylphenidate (Ritalin) can produce similar signs and symptoms, but in addition extremely high body temperatures can be found. Heroin intoxication presents with a depressed level of consciousness, decreased respirations, and pinpoint pupils. PCP can cause hallucinations as well as seizures, coma, and death. Other effects are nausea, vomiting, blurred vision, nystagmus, drooling, loss of balance, and dizziness. High doses can also cause delusions, paranoia, disordered thinking, and catatonia. Speech is often sparse and garbled. LSD intoxication can cause hallucinations or "bad trips." Massive doses can cause coma, respiratory arrest, vomiting, and hyperthermia.

130. The answer is e. (*Kaplan and Sadock, pp 101-102.*) The patient presents with a classic case of galactorrhea, caused by the blockade of dopamine receptors in the tuberoinfundibular tract. This blockade eliminates the inhibitory effect of dopamine on the release of prolactin from the anterior pituitary. With the inhibitory effect gone, patients on dopamine receptor antagonists can have a threefold rise in prolactin levels, leading to galactorrhea.

131. The answer is a. (*Kaplan and Sadock, p 129.*) In the case of hereditary Alzheimer disease that appears between the ages of 40 and 50, the *presenilin 1* gene, located on chromosome 14, is involved in 70% to 80% of cases. Another 20% to 30% are attributable to the *presenilin 2* gene, located on chromosome 1, responsible for heritable cases of Alzheimer disease appearing at age 50. A final 2% to 3% of Alzheimer cases, which appear after the age of 50, are attributable to the *β-amyloid precursor protein (APP)* gene located on chromosome 21.

132. The answer is c. *(Kaplan and Sadock, p 102.)* The dopaminergic system is thought to be involved in the brain's "reward system," and this involvement is thought to explain the very high addiction potential with regard to cocaine. "Knockout mice," in which the *dopamine transporter* gene has been deleted, respond neither biochemically nor behaviorally to cocaine.

133. The answer is b. *(Kaplan and Sadock, pp 520-521.)* Partial complex seizures usually (90% of the time) originate in the temporal lobe. Auras that consist of unpleasant odors often originate in the uncus, an area at the tip of the temporal lobe that is involved in processing olfactory sensations. In the past, such seizures were called uncinate fits.

134. The answer is e. *(Kaplan and Sadock, pp 766-767.)* Night terrors are characterized by a partial awakening accompanied by screaming, thrashing, and autonomic arousal. They are non-REM sleep events. Increase in blood pressure and heart rate, penile erection, and dreaming are associated with REM sleep.

135. The answer is a. *(Kaplan and Sadock, p 901.)* Diminished central serotonin has some role in suicidal behavior. Low concentrations of 5-HIAA have been associated with suicidal behavior, and 5-HIAA is a serotonin metabolite. This finding has been replicated in many studies. Low concentrations of 5-HIAA in the cerebrospinal fluid (CSF) also predicts the presence of future suicidal behavior.

136. The answer is e. *(Kaplan and Sadock, pp 604-605.)* It has been proven that a dysfunction of serotoninergic pathways is implicated in the genesis of obsessive-compulsive disorder. This finding is supported by the antiobsessional effects of medications, such as selective serotonin reuptake inhibitors (SSRIs) and clomipramine (a tricyclic), that increase the concentration of serotonin in the synaptic cleft. Of the other neurotransmitters, dopamine is linked to psychosis, acetylcholine plays a role in cognitive functions and memory, and norepinephrine is involved in anxiety disorders.

137. The answer is a. *(Kaplan and Sadock, pp 1041-1042.)* Hallucinations are the most common side effect of anti-Parkinson medications. Hallucinations occur in 30% of the treated patients and can be induced by any type of medication used to treat Parkinson disease, including dopaminergic agents such as L-dopa, ropinirole and amantidine, MAO inhibitors, and anticholinergic medications. The hallucinations usually consist of clear images of people and animals and may be preceded by sleep disturbances. Increasing age, polypharmacy, long treatment, and use of anticholinergic medications increase the risk for developing hallucinations. Reducing the dosage or eliminating anticholinergic agents is usually the only necessary treatment.

138. The answer is d. (*Kaplan and Sadock, p 107.*) Acetylcholine is most commonly associated with dementia of the Alzheimer type, as well as with other dementias. Anticholinergic agents in general have been known to impair learning and memory in normal people.

139 to 141. The answers are 139-c, 140-e, 141-a. (*Kaplan and Sadock, pp 98-110.*) CNS neurotransmitters include amino acids, biogenic amines, and neuropeptides. There are many other neurotransmitter substances, and many are still poorly understood. This is one of the most exciting areas of current psychiatric research. As more and more knowledge accrues, it becomes possible to develop more specific psychopharmacologic interventions. Glutamic and aspartic acids have excitatory properties. GABA is the principal inhibitory neurotransmitter. The biogenic amines include the catecholamines such as dopamine, norepinephrine, epinephrine, histamine, and the indolamine serotonin. Neuropeptides include β-endorphin, somatostatin, vasopressin, and substance P. Serotonin is affected primarily by fluoxetine, as it is a serotonin-specific reuptake inhibitor. Norepinephrine is affected by a wide array of the classical antidepressant drugs as well as some of the newer drugs like mirtazapine. Substance P is known to mediate the perception of pain, and neuropeptide Y has been shown to stimulate the appetite, making it an area of interest for obesity researchers.

142 and 143. The answers are 142-b, 143-a. (*Kaplan and Sadock, p 85.*) The localization of Broca and Wernicke aphasias are in the left hemisphere in their respective named areas (Broca area in the left inferior frontal lobe and Wernicke area in the left superior temporal lobe). Damage in the Wernicke area gives an aphasia which is characterized by fluent spontaneous speech, poor auditory comprehension, poor repetition ability, and poor naming ability. Damage in the Broca area gives an aphasia that is characterized by nonfluent spontaneous speech, good auditory comprehension, poor repetition ability, and poor naming ability. Conduction aphasia occurs in the left arcuate fasciculus region, and gives fluent spontaneous speech, good auditory comprehension, and poor repetition and naming. A global aphasia occurs from damage to the left perisylvian region, and as the name suggests, gives a nonfluent aphasia with poor auditory comprehension, repetition, and naming. An anomic aphasia occurs in the left angular gyrus, and affected individuals have fluent spontaneous speech, good auditory comprehension and repetition, and poor naming.

144. The answer is d. *(Kaplan and Sadock, p 881.)* Data from a series of animal experiments suggest that the hippocampus is the site for formation and storage of immediate and recent memories. It is even thought (though no data yet support this) that the hippocampal map is inappropriately reactivated during a déjà vu experience.

145. The answer is b. *(Kaplan and Sadock, p 871.)* Within the diencephalon, the dorsal medial nucleus of the thalamus and the mammillary bodies appear necessary for memory formation. These two structures are damaged in thiamine-deficient states usually seen in chronic alcoholics, and their inactivation is associated with Korsakoff syndrome.

146. The answer is a. *(Kaplan and Sadock, pp 111, 333.)* A family history of a similar disorder, choreiform movements as described, and the onset of a dementia-like illness with depression and apathy, make the diagnosis of Huntington chorea very likely. Patients with Huntington typically show atrophy of the caudate nucleus. The disorder is transmitted through a dominant gene. Symptoms typically do not occur until the age of 35 or later (the earlier the disease manifests, the more severe the disease tends to be).

147. The answer is b. *(Kaplan and Sadock, p 89.)* A lesion to the right prefrontal area may produce laughter, euphoria, and a tendency to joke and make puns. In contrast, a lesion to the left prefrontal area abolishes the normal mood-elevating influences of this area and produces depression and uncontrollable crying.

148. The answer is a. *(Kaplan and Sadock, pp 90-91.)* Dysfunction of the orbitofrontal area causes disinhibition, irritability, lability, euphoria, and lack of remorse. Insight and judgment are impaired; patients are distractible. These features are reminiscent of the diagnoses of antisocial personality disorder, intermittent explosive disorder, and episodic dyscontrol syndrome.

149. The answer is b. (*Kaplan and Sadock, pp 90-91.*) Lesions in the dorsolateral area lead to deficiencies of planning, monitoring, flexibility, and motivation. Patients may be unable to use foresight and feedback or to maintain goal-directedness, focus, or sustained effort. They appear inattentive and undermotivated, cannot plan novel cognitive activity, and exhibit a tendency to linger on trivial thoughts. They may echo the examiner's questions and react primarily to details of environmental stimuli—missing the forest for the trees.

150. The answer is e. (*Kaplan and Sadock, p 100.*) The caudate nucleus plays an important role in the modulation of motor acts. When functioning properly, the caudate acts as a gatekeeper to allow the motor system to perform only those acts that are goal directed. When it fails, extraneous acts are performed. The caudate shrinks dramatically in Huntington disease. The disorder is characterized by rigidity and gradually superimposed choreiform, or "dancing," movements.

151 to 156. The answers are 151-c, 152-e, 153-d, 154-a, 155-f, 156-b. (*Kaplan and Sadock, p 844.*) Vitamin deficiencies (and more rarely, their excess) can cause psychiatric symptoms. Patients with celiac disease, on kidney dialysis, who are heavy smokers, or who are pregnant are more at risk for folic acid deficiency, which can cause depression and dementia, in addition to neural tube defects in infants born to mothers with such deficits. Thiamine deficiency is rarely seen in industrialized society, but the acute depletion of already low stores of thiamine in an alcoholic patient may lead to Wernicke encephalopathy (think COAT: Confusion, Ophthalmoplegia, Ataxia, and Thiamine to treat) and Korsakoff syndrome (think RACK: Retrograde and Anterograde amnesia, Confabulation, Korsakoff syndrome). Vitamin B_{12} deficiency is most commonly found in the elderly, those status post gastric surgery, or in malnourished depressed patients. The most common psychiatric symptoms displayed in vitamin B_{12} deficiency include apathy, depressed mood, confusion, and memory deficits. A variety of neurologic deficits may coexist as well, among them, sensory deficits and the decrease or absence of deep tendon reflexes. Excesses of vitamins are generally seen in those who take massive doses of oral supplements, and the symptoms seen usually rapidly reverse once the supplements are removed. Vitamin A excess reveals itself with a yellowing of the skin and conjunctivae similar in some respects to jaundice. Vitamin D excess leads to the calcification of bone and soft tissue, as well as the formation of kidney stones (from hypercalcemia). Kidney damage that occurs may be irreversible. Vitamin E excess leads to problems with clotting, and if severe, may lead to hemorrhagic strokes. If necessary, vitamin K can help stop the bleeding. Vitamin E is often taken by patients in the belief that it provides protection against heart attacks, though there is no evidence to support this notion.

157 to 163. The answers are 157-c, 158-f, 159-g, 160-a, 161-b, 162-d, 163-e *(Kaplan and Sadock, p 105.)* At least 14 distinct serotonin receptors have now been recognized. The fact that they are distributed throughout the body means they are sometimes responsible for a whole host of side effects when serotonergic drugs are used. Receptors in the limbic system may cause an initial increase in anxiety after being started on a serotinergic drug. Receptors in the intestines (90% of the body's serotonin is found in the intestines!) may cause gastrointestinal (GI) upset and diarrhea. Receptors in the cranial blood vessels may cause headache. Receptors in the basal ganglia may be responsible for akathisia and agitation. Receptors in either the brain stem vomiting center (area postrema) or the hypothalamus may cause nausea and vomiting. Receptors in the various parts of the brain stem's sleep centers may cause either insomnia or somnolence. Receptors in the spinal cord pathways may cause sexual dysfunction. It is very difficult and near to impossible to predict which side effects will occur in a particular patient when serotonergic drugs are used.

164 to 168. The answers are 164-c, 165-d, 166-a, 167-b, 168-e. *(Kaplan and Sadock, pp 110-111.)* MRIs distinguish between white and gray matter better than CT scans, and allow one to see smaller lesions, as well as white matter abnormalities. Chronic infections, including neurosyphilis, may produce a characteristic enhancement of the meninges at the base of the brain. (Other chronic infections such as cryptococcosis, tuberculosis, and Lyme disease, may also produce this kind of finding.) Dementia and a gait disorder in a 40-year-old woman brings the diagnosis of normal pressure hydrocephalus to the forefront. The MRI in this case would show a dilatation of the ventricles. The 36-year-old man in question 166 has multiple sclerosis; his MRI would show periventricular patches of increased signal intensity. These are the multiple sclerosis plaques. The 40-year-old man in question 167 has Huntington disease, which produces a characteristic appearance on MRI of atrophy of the caudate nucleus. The 72-year-old woman in question 168 has a dementia. The appearance of patches of increased signal in the white matter (not just periventricular in location) would give the diagnosis of a vascular dementia.

169 to 172. The answers are 169-a, 170-b, 171-c, 172-d (*Kaplan and Sadock, p 118.*) The four basic EEG wave forms are alpha, beta, delta, and theta. Alpha is the frequency range from 8 to 13 Hz. It emerges with closing of the eyes and with relaxation, and attenuates with eye opening or mental exertion.

Beta is the frequency range from 13 Hz to about 30 Hz. It is seen usually on both sides in symmetrical distribution and is most evident frontally. Beta activity is closely linked to motor behavior and is generally attenuated during active movements. Low-amplitude beta with multiple and varying frequencies is often associated with active, busy, or anxious thinking and active concentration. Rhythmic beta with a dominant set of frequencies is associated with various pathologies and drug effects, especially benzodiazepines. It may be absent or reduced in areas of cortical damage. It is the dominant rhythm in patients who are alert or anxious or who have their eyes open.

Delta is the frequency range up to 3.5 to 4 Hz. It tends to be the highest in amplitude and the slowest waves. It is seen normally in adults in slow wave sleep. It is also seen normally in babies. It may occur focally with subcortical lesions and in general distribution with diffuse lesions, metabolic encephalopathy hydrocephalus, or deep midline lesions.

Theta is the frequency range from 4 to 7 Hz. Theta is seen normally in young children. It may be seen in drowsiness or arousal in older children and adults; it can also be seen in meditation. Excess theta for age represents abnormal activity. This range has been associated with reports of relaxed, meditative, and creative states.

Disorders of Childhood and Adolescence

Questions

173. A 5-year-old boy is brought to the psychiatrist because he has difficulty paying attention in school. He fidgets and squirms and will not stay seated in class. It is noted that at home he talks excessively and has difficulty waiting for his turn. His language and motor skills are appropriate for his age. Which of the following is the most likely diagnosis?

a. Oppositional defiant disorder (ODD)
b. Attention-deficit hyperactivity disorder (ADHD)
c. Pervasive developmental disorder
d. Separation anxiety disorder
e. Mild mental retardation

174. In the case described above, what other criteria *must* be present in order for this diagnosis to be met?

a. The child often loses things necessary for tasks or activities (toys, school assignments).
b. The symptoms must have been present for at least 6 months.
c. The symptoms must be present in at least 3 separate settings.
d. The child often blurts out answers before questions have been completed.
e. There must be clear evidence of clinically significant impairment in social functioning.

175. A 4-year-old girl is brought to her pediatrician because her parents think she does not seem to be "developing normally." The girl's mother states that her daughter seemed normal for at least the first 2 to 3 years of her life. She was walking and beginning to speak in sentences. She was able to play with her mother and older sister. The mother has been noticing that over the past 2 months her daughter has lost these previously acquired abilities. She will no longer play with anyone else and has stopped speaking entirely. She has lost all bowel control, when previously she had not needed a diaper for at least a year. Which of the following is the most likely diagnosis?

a. Rett disorder
b. Childhood disintegrative disorder
c. Autism
d. Asperger disorder
e. Pervasive developmental disorder

176. The parents of an 8-year-old boy with a normal IQ are concerned because he is a very slow reader and does not appear to understand what he reads. When the boy reads aloud, he misses words and changes the sequence of the letters. They also note that he has problems with spelling, though he is otherwise quite creative in his ability to write stories. On examination, the child displays verbal language defects as well, though primarily he communicates clearly. His hearing and vision are normal and he has no trouble with motor skills. Which of the following is the most likely diagnosis for this child?

a. Developmental expressive writing disorder
b. Dyslexia
c. Developmental articulation disorder
d. Pervasive developmental disorder
e. Developmental coordination disorder

177. A 13-year-old boy is brought to the emergency room by his parents after he set fire to their home. He has been seen in the emergency room on multiple occasions for a variety of symptoms, including suicidality, homicidality, uncontrollable tantrums, and pica. Of those symptoms, which is most commonly seen in adolescents when seen by psychiatrists in the emergency room?

a. Arson
b. Suicidality
c. Homicidality
d. Uncontrollable tantrums
e. Pica

178. A 5-year-old is being evaluated for ADHD. He has a past history of failure to thrive and he is still at the 15th percentile for weight and height. The evaluator notices that he has unusually small eyes with short palpebral fissures, as well as a thin upper lip with a smooth philtrum. Which substance did his mother most likely abuse during pregnancy?

a. Heroin
b. Nicotine
c. Cannabis
d. Alcohol
e. Cocaine

179. A 7-year-old boy avoids sleepovers because he wets his bed 1 to 2 times per week and is afraid his friends would tease him. He has never achieved a year-long period of dryness throughout the night. A physiologic work-up shows no evidence of an organic cause for this problem, and there is no evidence of a psychiatric disorder in any other category. Which of the following treatments is likely to be effective and should be tried first?

a. Pharmacotherapy with imipramine
b. Bladder training (reward for delaying micturition during daylight hours)
c. Classic conditioning with a bell-and-pad apparatus
d. Pharmacotherapy with desmopressin
e. Psychotherapy

180. A 13-year-old girl grunts and clears her throat several times in an hour, and her conversation is often interrupted by random shouting. She also performs idiosyncratic, complex motor activities such as turning her head to the right while she shuts her eyes and opens her mouth. She can prevent these movements for brief periods of time, with effort. Which of the following is the most appropriate treatment for this disorder?

a. Individual psychodynamic psychotherapy
b. Lorazepam
c. Methylphenidate
d. Haloperidol
e. Imipramine

181. A 6-year-old boy has been diagnosed with ADHD and started on Ritalin. About which of the following serious side effects should the child psychiatrist warn the boy's parents?

a. Tics
b. Cardiac conduction abnormalities
c. Choreiform movements
d. Leukopenia
e. Hepatitis

182. Every morning on school days, an 8-year-old girl becomes tearful and distressed and claims she feels sick. Once in school, she often goes to the nurse, complaining of headaches and stomach pains. At least once a week, she misses school or is picked up early by her mother due to her complaints. Her pediatrician has ruled out organic causes for the physical symptoms. The child is usually symptom free on weekends, unless her parents go out and leave her with a babysitter. Which of the following is the most likely diagnosis?

a. Separation anxiety disorder
b. Major depression
c. Somatization disorder
d. Generalized anxiety disorder
e. Reactive attachment disorder

183. A 1-year-old girl has been hospitalized on numerous occasions for periods of apnea. Each time, her mother called an ambulance after her daughter had suddenly stopped breathing. All work-ups in the hospital have been negative, and the patient has never had an episode in front of anyone but her mother. The patient's mother seems very involved with the child and the staff on the unit, and she does not seem hesitant about consenting to lab tests on her daughter, even if the tests are invasive. Which of the following psychiatric disorders (in the mother) must be considered in this case?

a. Panic disorder
b. Generalized anxiety disorder
c. Factitious disorder (by proxy)
d. Malingering
e. Separation anxiety disorder

184. A social worker makes a routine visit to a 3-year-old boy who has just been returned to his biological mother after spending 3 months in foster care as a result of severe neglect. The child initially appears very shy and clings fearfully to his mother. Later on, he starts playing in a very destructive and disorganized way. When the mother tries to stop him from throwing blocks at her, he starts kicking and biting. The mother becomes enraged and starts shouting. Which of the following is the most likely diagnosis for this child?

a. Oppositional defiant disorder
b. ADHD
c. Reactive attachment disorder
d. Posttraumatic stress disorder (PTSD)
e. Major depression

185. A first-grade teacher is concerned about a 6-year-old girl in her class who has not spoken a single word since school started. The little girl participates appropriately in the class activities and uses gestures and drawings and nods and shakes her head to communicate. The parents report that the little girl talks only in the home and only in the presence of her closest relatives. Which of the following is the most likely diagnosis?

a. Autism
b. Expressive language disorder
c. Oppositional defiant disorder
d. School phobia
e. Selective mutism

186. A 4-year-old boy is brought to the physician by his parents because he experiences episodes of waking in the middle of the night and screaming. The parents state that when they get to the boy's room during one of these episodes, they find him in his bed, thrashing wildly, his eyes wide open. He pushes them away when they try to comfort him. After 2 minutes, the boy suddenly falls asleep, and the next day he has no memory of the episode. Which of the following medications should be the first choice to treat this disorder?

a. Haloperidol
b. Diazepam
c. Methylphenidate
d. Amitriptyline
e. Valproic acid

187. A 14-year-old boy is brought to the physician because he told his mother he wished he were dead. He has been irritable for the past several weeks, and has been isolating himself in his room, avoiding his friends. He has been complaining of general aches and pains as well. Which of the following symptoms may well also be present in this patient?

a. Hyperactivity
b. Fire-setting
c. Homicidal ideation
d. Presence of a hallucination
e. Obsession about cleanliness

188. A 12-year-old boy is brought to the psychiatrist because his mother says the boy is driving her "nuts." She reports that he constantly argues with her and his father, does not follow any of the house rules, and incessantly teases his sister. She says that he is spiteful and vindictive and loses his temper easily. Once he is mad, he stays that way for long periods of time. The mother notes that the boy started this behavior only about 1 year previously. While she states that this behavior started at home, it has now spread to school, where his grades are dropping because he refuses to participate. The patient maintains that none of this is his fault—his parents are simply being unreasonable. He denies feeling depressed and notes that he sleeps well through the night. Which of the following is the most likely diagnosis?

a. Oppositional defiant disorder (ODD)
b. Antisocial personality disorder
c. Conduct disorder
d. Childhood-onset schizophrenia
e. Mania

189. A 5-year-old boy shows no interest in other children and ignores adults other than his parents. He spends hours lining up his toy cars or spinning their wheels but does not use them for "make-believe" play. He rarely uses speech to communicate, and his parents state that he has never done so. Physical examination indicates that his head is of normal circumference and his gait is normal. Which of the following is the most likely diagnosis for this boy?

a. Obsessive-compulsive disorder
b. Asperger syndrome
c. Childhood disintegrative disorder
d. Autism
e. Rett disorder

Disorders of Childhood and Adolescence

Answers

173. The answer is b. (*Kaplan and Sadock, pp 1214-1215.*) Excessive motor activity, usually with intrusive and annoying qualities, poor sustained attention, difficulties inhibiting impulsive behaviors in social situations and on cognitive tasks, and difficulties with peers are the main characteristics of ADHD, combined type. Symptoms must be present in two or more settings (in this case, home and school) and must cause significant impairment.

174. The answer is b. (*Kaplan and Sadock, p 1208.*) For a diagnosis of ADHD, symptoms must be present for at least 6 months in at least two settings. While clinically significant impairment must exist for the disorder to be diagnosed, it can occur in social, academic, *or* occupational functioning (it does not have to occur in social functioning alone). Six or more symptoms of inattention (including losing things necessary for tasks or activities) *or* six or more symptoms of hyperactivity-impulsivity (including blurting out answers before questions have been completed) must be present for the diagnosis to be made.

175. The answer is b. (*Kaplan and Sadock, pp 1200-1201.*) Childhood disintegrative disorder is characterized by apparently normal development through at least the first 2 years of life. During this time, age-appropriate skills such as verbal and nonverbal communication, social relationships, bowel and bladder control, and play, all develop normally. The disease manifests itself as a clinically significant loss of previously acquired skills before the age of 10. In Rett disorder, the onset of the disease occurs earlier, usually 6 months after birth, and there are characteristic hand stereotypies that do not occur in childhood disintegrative disorder. The presence of the apparently normal development of speech and other behaviors, followed by the loss of these, distinguishes this disorder from autism, Asperger disorder, and pervasive developmental disorder, where there is no loss of previously acquired skills.

176. The answer is b. (*Moore and Jefferson, pp 33-34.*) Dyslexia occurs in 3% to 10% of the population. When a reading disorder is caused by a defect in visual or hearing acuity, it is excluded by diagnostic criteria from being a developmental reading disorder. Almost all patients with this problem have spelling difficulties, and nearly all have verbal language defects. Children do not grow out of the disorder by adulthood. It is believed that the most common etiology relates to cortical brain pathology. The child in this question is able to read and attend school; thus, he cannot have pervasive developmental disorder. His ability to write stories and communicate primarily clearly and his normal motor skills rule out the other diagnoses listed. Dyslexia is a common comorbid finding with those diagnosed with ADHD.

177. The answer is b. (*Kaplan and Sadock, p 919.*) Suicidal behavior is the most common reason for a psychiatrist to see an adolescent in an emergency room setting. Important in the evaluation of these children is an assessment of the stability and supportiveness of the home environment, and the care-giver's competence in taking care of the adolescent. These factors will figure in to a clinician's decision as to whether a potentially suicidal adolescent must be admitted to an inpatient unit or may be released home to be closely monitored.

178. The answer is d. (*Jacobson and Jacobson, pp 352-353,357.*) Fetal alcohol syndrome occurs in 1 to 2 live births per 1000, and among 2% to 10% of alcoholic mothers. Fetal alcohol syndrome is characterized by intrauterine growth retardation and persistent postnatal poor growth, microcephaly, developmental delays, attentional deficits, learning disabilities, and hyperactivity. Characteristic facial features are microphthalmia with short palpebral fissures, midface hypoplasia, thin upper lip, and a smooth and/or long philtrum. Children whose mothers used opiates during pregnancy are born passively addicted to the drugs and exhibit withdrawal symptoms in the first days and weeks of life. During the first year of life, these infants show poor motor coordination, hyperactivity, and inattention. These problems persist during school-age years, although few differences in cognitive performance are reported. Infants exposed to cannabis prenatally present with decreased visual responsiveness, tremor, increased startle reflex, and disrupted sleep patterns. Long-term longitudinal outcome studies are few and contradictory. Prenatal exposure to cocaine causes impaired startle response; impaired habituation, recognition, and reactivity to novel stimuli;

and increased irritability in infants. Older children present with language delays, poor motor coordination, hyperactivity, and attentional deficits.

179. The answer is c. *(Kaplan and Sadock, pp 1247-1248.)* This child has enuresis of a nonorganic type (he had a negative organic work-up). Nocturnal enuresis is not diagnosed before age 5, an age at which continence is usually expected. The incidence in boys is somewhat higher than in girls. This disorder is often associated with daytime (diurnal) wetting. Nocturnal enuresis usually is diagnosed in childhood, although adolescent onset does occur. The treatment of choice for enuresis is the use of classic conditioning with a bell (or buzzer) and a pad. This is generally the most effective treatment, with success in over 50% of all cases. Successful responses with this treatment also tend to be maintained over time. It also does not have the side effects of the pharmacotherapies. Bladder training, while sometimes effective, is decidedly less so than the bell and pad. Likewise, psychotherapy has not been shown to be effective in treating this disorder, though it may be helpful in dealing with the emotional difficulties that arise secondary to the disorder.

180. The answer is d. *(Jacobson and Jacobson, pp 87-88.)* Vocal tics such as grunting, barking, throat clearing, coprolalia (the repetitive speaking of vulgarities), shouting, and simple and complex motor tics are characteristic of Tourette syndrome. Pharmacological treatment of this disorder includes neuroleptics and α_2 agonists (clonidine, guanfacine).

181. The answer is a. *(Moore and Jefferson, pp 505-506.)* Common side effects of methylphenidate include loss of appetite and weight, irritability, oversensitivity and crying spells, headaches, and abdominal pain. Insomnia may occur, particularly when this agent is dispensed late in the day. Tics, while a less frequent complication of stimulant treatment, can cause significant impairment. (Whether this is the drug causing tics or the unmasking of a previous tic predisposition is unclear.) Choreiform movements and night terrors are side effects of another stimulant, pemoline. Leukopenia, hepatitis, and cardiac arrhythmias are not associated with stimulant treatment.

182. The answer is a. *(Jefferson and Moore, pp 52-53.)* Separation anxiety disorder is characterized by manifestations of distress when the child has to be separated from loved ones. The distress often leads to school refusal, refusal to sleep alone, multiple somatic symptoms, and complaints when the child is separated from loved ones, and at times may be associated with full-blown panic attacks. The child is typically afraid that harm will come either to loved ones or to him- or herself during the time of separation. This is normal behavior in children 1 to 3 years old, after which it is thought to be pathological. Reactive attachment disorder is seen in infancy or early childhood. The child shows either excessively inhibited or disinhibited attachments—inappropriate social relatedness—as a result of grossly impaired caregiving. Reactive attachment disorder is characterized by markedly disturbed and developmentally inappropriate ways of relating socially in most contexts. It can take the form of a persistent failure to initiate or respond to most social interactions in a developmentally appropriate way—known as the "inhibited" form—or can present itself as indiscriminate sociability, such as excessive familiarity with relative strangers—known as the "disinhibited form."

183. The answer is c. *(Jacobson and Jacobson, p 472.)* In factitious disorder (Munchausen syndrome) by proxy, a caregiver, usually the mother, fabricates or produces symptoms of illness in a child. The caregiver's motive is to vicariously receive care and attention from health providers through the sick child. The severity of the disorder varies from cases in which symptoms are completely fabricated to cases in which the mother causes serious physical harm to or even the death of the child. Mothers in cases of Munchausen by proxy are extremely attentive to their children and often are considered model parents. These mothers are not cognitively impaired or psychotic; on the contrary, they are often quite accomplished and knowledgeable and frequently work or have worked in the medical field. Not infrequently, more than one child is victimized in a family, particularly in cases of suffocation disguised as sudden infant death syndrome (SIDS) or apnea. A very pathological relationship develops between the mother and the victimized child, to the point that older children often collude with the mother in producing the symptoms.

184. The answer is c. *(Kaplan and Sadock, pp 1250-1251.)* Reactive attachment disorder is the product of a severely dysfunctional early relationship between the principal caregiver and the child. When caregivers consistently disregard the child's physical or emotional needs, the child fails to develop a secure and stable attachment with them. This failure causes a severe disturbance of the child's ability to relate to others, manifested in a variety of behavioral and interpersonal problems. Some children are fearful, inhibited, withdrawn, and apathetic; others are aggressive, disruptive, and disorganized, with low frustration tolerance and poor affect modulation. This condition is often confused with ODD or ADHD.

185. The answer is e. *(Kaplan and Sadock, pp 1286-1287.)* In selective mutism, a child voluntarily abstains from talking in particular situations (usually at school) while remaining appropriately verbal at home. Some children speak only with their parents and siblings and are mute with relatives and friends. Children with selective mutism do not have a language impediment, nor do they display the lack of social interactions, lack of imagination, and stereotyped behavior characteristic of autism. On the contrary, they can be quite interactive and communicative in a nonverbal way, using drawing, writing, and pantomime. Children with school phobia refuse to go to school but do not have problems communicating through language. Oppositional defiant disorder is characterized by persistent refusal to follow rules and defiance toward authorities, not by failure to speak.

186. The answer is b. *(Kaplan and Sadock, pp 766-767.)* The child in the question is experiencing episodes of sleep terror disorder, a dyssomnia characterized by sudden partial arousal accompanied by piercing screams, motor agitation, disorientation, and autonomic arousal. The episodes take place during the transition from deep sleep to REM sleep. Children do not report nightmares (which would be associated with REM sleep) and do not have any memory of the episodes the next day. Sleep terrors occur in 3% of children and 1% of adults. Although specific treatment for this disorder is seldom required, in rare cases it is necessary. Diazepam (Valium) in small doses at bedtime improves the condition and sometimes completely eliminates the attacks.

187. The answer is d. *(Kaplan and Sadock, pp 1259-1260.)* The child in question is suffering from a major depressive disorder. Depressive disorders are not rare in children, and often children with depression have relatives who also suffer from depression or another mood disorder. The incidence of depression is estimated to be 0.9% in preschoolers, 1.9% in school-age children, and 4.7% in adolescents. The incidence is considerably higher among children with neurological or medical illnesses. The diagnosis can be difficult because younger children's symptoms differ from the symptoms of depression usually displayed by adults. Often, aggression and irritability replace sad affect, and poor school functioning or refusal to go to school may be the prominent manifestations. Psychotic symptoms are present in one-third of the cases of childhood major depression.

188. The answer is a. (*Kaplan and Sadock, pp 1219-1220.*) This patient has oppositional defiant disorder. The presence of the symptoms, including being angry, spiteful and vindictive, losing his temper quickly, and deliberately annoying others, for at least 6 months is characteristic of the disease. It is also characteristic that the boy denies that he has a problem, blaming it instead on others. While sometimes the behavior starts outside the home, other times, as in this question, the disorder starts at home and then is carried to school and other arenas. This patient has no history of aggressive behavior toward animals or others and has not been destructive or in trouble with the law, making conduct disorder less likely. He is under the age of 18, the minimum age for which antisocial personality disorder may be diagnosed. He denies mood symptoms and is sleeping well through the night, making mania unlikely. No psychotic symptoms were noted, ruling out childhood schizophrenia.

189. The answer is d. (*Jacobson and Jacobson, pp 295-302.*) Autistic disorder is characterized by lack of interest in social interactions, severely impaired verbal and nonverbal communication, stereotyped behaviors, and a very restricted range of interests. Children with autism do not involve themselves in imaginative and imitative play and can spend hours lining and spinning things or dismantling toys and putting them together. Patients with obsessive-compulsive disorder may spend hours on repetitive tasks (such as lining up toys) but do not show the difficulties with language and social interaction that this patient displays. Patients with Asperger syndrome show no clinically significant delay in spoken or receptive language development, making this diagnosis unlikely. Patients with childhood disintegrative disorder have approximately a 2-year period of normal development (including speech and interpersonal skills) before this regresses; this patient has never apparently had such a period. Patients with Rett disorder by the age of 5 would be expected to have microcephaly and a disordered gait (unsteady and stiff).

Cognitive Disorders and Consultation-Liaison Psychiatry

Questions

190. For the past 10 years, the memory of a 74-year-old woman has progressively declined. Lately, she has caused several small kitchen fires by forgetting to turn off the stove, she cannot remember how to cook her favorite recipes, and she becomes disoriented and confused at night. She identifies an increasing number of objects as "that thing" because she cannot recall the correct name. Her muscle strength and balance are intact. Which of the following is the most likely diagnosis?

a. Huntington disease
b. Multi-infarct dementia
c. Creutzfeldt-Jakob disease
d. Alzheimer disease
e. Wilson disease

191. A 70-year-old man with a dementing disorder dies in a car accident. During the previous 5 years, his personality had dramatically changed and he had caused much embarrassment to his family because of his intrusive and inappropriate behavior. Pathological examination of his brain shows frontotemporal atrophy, gliosis of the frontal lobes' white matter, characteristic intracellular inclusions, and swollen neurons. Amyloid plaques and neurofibrillary tangles are absent. Which of the following is the most likely diagnosis?

a. Alzheimer disease
b. Pick disease
c. Creutzfeldt-Jakob disease
d. Vitamin B_{12} deficiency dementia
e. HIV dementia

192. A 69-year-old woman slips on the ice and hits her head on the pavement. During the following 3 weeks, she develops a persistent headache, is increasingly distractible and forgetful, and becomes fearful and disoriented at night. Which of the following is the most likely cause of these changes?

a. Subdural hematoma
b. Frontal lobe meningioma
c. Korsakoff disease
d. Epidural hematoma
e. Multi-infarct dementia

193. A 43-year-old man is admitted to the neurology service after he went blind suddenly on the morning of admission. The patient does not seem overly concerned with his sudden lack of vision. The only time he gets upset during the interview is when he is discussing his mother's recent death in Mexico—he was supposed to bring his mother to the United States, but did not because he had been using drugs and did not save the necessary money. Physical examination is completely negative. Which of the following is the most likely diagnosis?

a. Conversion disorder
b. Hypochondriasis
c. Factitious disorder
d. Malingering
e. Delusional disorder

194. A 76-year-old woman was admitted to the hospital after she was found lying on the floor of her bedroom by her daughter. In the hospital, the patient was found to be incoherent. She was also hypervigilant and had disorganized thoughts. The woman's medications before hospitalization included digoxin and a benzodiazepine, which had been recently started because the patient had been complaining of insomnia. What is the most likely diagnosis?

a. Delirium secondary to a general medical condition
b. Delirium secondary to substance intoxication
c. Dementia of the Alzheimer type
d. Vascular dementia
e. Pseudodementia secondary to major depression

195. A 24-year-old man smells burnt rubber, then turns his head and upper body to the right, makes chewing movements, and fumbles with his clothes. During the episode, which lasts 1 minute, he appears dazed. Which of the following is the most likely diagnosis?

a. Frontal lobe tumor
b. Derealization disorder
c. Conversion disorder
d. Absence seizure
e. Partial complex seizure

196. A 55-year-old man comes to the physician with the chief complaint of daytime drowsiness. He states that although he goes to bed at 10 PM and doesn't get up until 6 AM, he is chronically tired and must take naps during the day. He wakes up in the morning with a headache and a dry mouth. His wife states that he snores loudly. Which of the following is the most likely diagnosis?

a. Obstructive sleep apnea
b. Narcolepsy
c. Central apnea
d. Recurrent hypersomnia
e. Major depression

197. A 24-year-old woman is hospitalized after a suicide gesture during which she superficially slashed both her wrists. At the team meeting 3 days later, the male resident argues that the patient has been doing quite well, seems to be responding to therapy, and should be allowed to leave on a pass. The nursing staff angrily argues that the resident is showing favoritism to the patient, and because of her poor compliance with the unit rules, she should not be allowed out. The resident insists the nurses are being punitive. The defense mechanism being used by the patient in this scenario is a feature of which of the following personality disorders?

a. Narcissistic
b. Histrionic
c. Borderline
d. Antisocial
e. Dependent

198. A 45-year-old woman, who has been in chronic medical treatment for her asthma, has thin arms and legs but has a large amount of fat deposited on her abdomen, chest, and shoulders. Her skin is thin and atrophic, and she bruises easily. She has purple striae on her abdomen. Physical examination shows elevated blood pressure and laboratory tests show decreased glucose tolerance. Which of the following psychiatric diagnoses is commonly present in a patient in such chronic treatment?

a. Major depression
b. Bipolar-mania
c. Substance-induced mood disorder
d. Delirium
e. Schizoaffective disorder

199. A 69-year-old man with a diagnosis of delirium has symptoms of psychosis that include: frightening auditory and visual hallucinations and paranoid delusions. Which of the following medications should be chosen first for this man's symptoms?

a. Haloperidol
b. Quetiapine
c. Diazepam (Valium)
d. Olanzepine
e. Ziprasidone

200. A 40-year-old woman's cognitive functions have progressively deteriorated for several years, to the point where she needs nursing home–level care. She is depressed, easily irritated, and prone to aggressive outbursts, a dramatic change from her premorbid personality. She also presents with irregular, purposeless, and asymmetrical movements of her face, limbs, and trunk, which worsen when she is upset and disappear in sleep. Her MRI shows atrophy of the caudal nucleus and the putamen. Which of the following is the most likely diagnosis of this patient?

a. Creutzfeldt-Jakob disease
b. Wilson disease
c. Huntington disease
d. Alzheimer disease
e. Multi-infarct dementia

201. A 37-year-old mildly retarded man with trisomy 21 syndrome has been increasingly forgetful. He has started to make frequent mistakes when counting change at the grocery store where he has worked for several years. In the past, he used to perform this task without difficulty. He often cannot recall the names of common objects, and he has started annoying customers with his intrusive questions. Which of the following is the most likely diagnosis of this patient?

a. Pseudodementia
b. Hypothalamic tumor
c. Alzheimer disease
d. Wilson disease
e. Thiamine deficiency

202. A 72-year-old retired English professor with a long history of hypertension has been having difficulties with tasks he used to find easy and enjoyable, such as crossword puzzles and letter writing, because he cannot remember the correct words and his handwriting has deteriorated. He has also been having difficulty remembering the events of previous days and he moves and thinks at a slower pace. These symptoms have been progressing slowly in a stepwise fashion over time. Subsequently, he develops slurred speech. Which of the following is the most likely diagnosis?

a. Multi-infarct dementia
b. German-Strausser syndrome
c. Rett disorder
d. Wernicke-Korsakoff syndrome
e. Alzheimer disease

203. A previously healthy 60-year-old man undergoes a corneal transplant. Three months later, he is profoundly demented, demonstrates myoclonic jerks on examination, and has an EEG that shows periodic bursts of electrical activity superimposed on a slow background. Which of the following is the most likely diagnosis?

a. Wilson disease
b. Multi-infarct dementia
c. Creutzfeldt-Jakob disease
d. Epilepsy
e. Pseudodementia

204. A 53-year-old man is admitted to the cardiac intensive care unit after a myocardial infarction. The day after he is admitted, when the physician enters the room, the patient loudly declares that he "feels fine" and proceeds to get down on the floor to demonstrate this assertion by doing pushups. Once persuaded to get back into bed, the patient becomes angry about the poor food quality and feels that only the "most qualified" specialist in the hospital should be treating him because he is, after all, the CEO of his own company. The patient's wife notes that this demanding behavior and haughty attitude are not unusual for him. Which of the following psychiatric diagnoses is most likely for this patient?

a. Mania
b. Acute psychotic disorder
c. Narcissistic personality disorder
d. Delusional disorder
e. Schizoaffective disorder

Questions 205 and 206

205. A 22-year-old college student comes to the physician with the complaint of shortness of breath during anxiety-provoking situations, such as examinations. She also notes perioral tingling, carpopedal spasms, and feelings of derealization at the same time. All of the symptoms pass after the anxiety over the situation has faded. The episodes have never occurred "out of the blue." Which of the following is the most likely diagnosis?

a. Panic disorder
b. Generalized anxiety disorder
c. Hyperventilation
d. Anxiety disorder not otherwise specified
e. Anxiety disorder secondary to a general medical condition

206. Which of the following treatments should the physician suggest first for the patient in the vignette above?

a. Alprazolam prn
b. Fluoxetine daily
c. Rebreathe into a paper bag during the episode
d. Biofeedback
e. Hypnosis

207. A 25-year-old woman is brought to the physician by her boyfriend after he noticed a change in her personality over the preceding 6 months. He states that she frequently becomes excessively preoccupied with a single theme, often religious in nature. She was not previously a religious person. He also notes that she often perseverates on a theme while she is speaking, and that she is overinclusive in her descriptions. Finally, he notes that while previously the two had a satisfying sexual life, now the patient appears to have no sex drive whatsoever. The physician finds the patient to be very emotionally intense as well. Physical examination was normal. Which of the following is the most likely diagnosis?

a. Wernicke-Korsakoff syndrome
b. Temporal lobe epilepsy
c. Pick disease
d. Multiple sclerosis
e. HIV-related dementia

208. A 23-year-old man comes to the physician with the complaint that his memory has worsened over the past 2 months and that he has difficulty concentrating. He has lost interest in his friends and his work. He has difficulty with abstract thoughts and problem solving. He has also felt depressed. MRI scan shows parenchymal abnormalities. Which of the following is the most likely diagnosis?

a. Alzheimer disease
b. Vascular dementia
c. HIV-related dementia
d. Lewy body disease
e. Binswanger disease

Questions 209 and 210

209. A 37-year-old alcoholic is brought to the emergency room after he was found unconscious in the street. He is hospitalized for dehydration and pneumonia. While being treated, he becomes acutely confused and agitated. He cannot move his eyes upward or to the right, and he is ataxic. Which of the following is the most likely diagnosis?

a. Alcohol intoxication
b. Korsakoff syndrome
c. Alcohol delirium
d. Wernicke encephalopathy
e. Alcohol seizures

210. Which of the following is the most appropriate treatment for the patient in the vignette above?

a. Dilantin
b. Valium
c. Haloperidol
d. Amobarbitol
e. Thiamine

211. A 65-year-old woman is brought to the physician because she has become easily distractible, apathetic, and unconcerned about her appearance. She has trouble remembering familiar words and locations, and she experiences urinary incontinence. On physical examination, her gait is seen to be ataxic. She does not exhibit any involuntary movements. When copying a complex picture, she makes many mistakes. The patient most likely has which of the following disorders?

a. Parkinson disease
b. Thiamine deficiency
c. Vitamin B_{12} deficiency
d. Wilson disease
e. Normal-pressure hydrocephalus

Questions 212 to 214

212. A 43-year-old woman comes to the emergency room with a temperature of 38.3°C (101°F) and a large suppurating ulcer on her left shoulder. This is the third such episode for this woman. Her physical examination is otherwise normal, except for the presence of multiple scars on her abdomen. Which of the following is the most likely diagnosis?

a. Malingering
b. Somatoform disorder
c. Borderline personality disorder
d. Factitious disorder
e. Body dysmorphic disorder

213. Which of the following etiologies is most likely underlying the behavior of the woman in the vignette above?

a. Primary gain
b. Secondary gain
c. Psychosis
d. Marginal intellectual function
e. Drug-seeking behavior

214. A 26-year-old man comes to the emergency room with the chief complaint of suicidal ideation. He is admitted to the psychiatric ward, where he is noncompliant with all treatment regimens and does not show any psychiatric symptoms other than his insistence that he is suicidal. It is subsequently discovered that he is wanted by the police, who have a warrant for his arrest. Which of the following best describes this behavior?

a. Primary gain
b. Secondary gain
c. Displacement
d. Rationalization
e. Marginal intellectual function

215. A 32-year-old woman who has a chronic psychiatric disorder, multiple medical problems, and alcoholism comes to the physician because her breasts have started leaking a whitish fluid. Which of the following endogenous substances is likely to have caused this phenomenon?

a. Estrogen
b. Thyroid hormone
c. Progesterone
d. Prolactin
e. Alcohol dehydrogenase

216. A 3-year-old child is brought to the emergency room by his parents after they found him having a generalized seizure at home. The child's breath smells of garlic, and he has bloody diarrhea, vomiting, and muscle twitching. Which of the following poisons is it likely that this child has encountered?

a. Thallium
b. Lead
c. Arsenic
d. Carbon monoxide
e. Aluminum

Questions 217 and 218

217. A 34-year-old woman comes to the physician with the chief complaint of abdominal pain. She states that she has been reading on the internet and is convinced that she has ovarian cancer. She says that she is particularly concerned because the other physicians she has seen for this pain have all told her that she does not have cancer, and she has been having the pain for over 8 months. She reports that she has undergone pelvic examinations, ultrasounds, and other diagnostic work-ups, all of which have been negative. She tells the physician that she is initially reassured by the negative tests, but then the pain returns and she becomes convinced that she has cancer again. She notes that she has taken so much time off from work in the past 8 months that she has been reprimanded by her boss. Which of the following is the most likely diagnosis?

a. Pain disorder
b. Malingering
c. Factitious disorder
d. Hypochondriasis
e. Conversion disorder

218. Which of the following courses of action is most likely to be helpful in the case of the woman in the vignette above?

a. Refer the patient to psychotherapy.
b. Start the patient on an antidepressant.
c. Have the patient see a primary care physician at regular intervals.
d. Begin a diagnostic work-up for ovarian cancer.
e. Start the patient on an antipsychotic for her delusional belief.

219. A man given a sugar pill for mild pain reports that 15 minutes later the pain has completely resolved. Which of the following conclusions is most appropriate about this occurrence?

a. The man is drug seeking.
b. The man is malingering.
c. The man has a factitious disorder.
d. The man is demonstrating a placebo response.
e. The man had no real pain to begin with.

220. A 53-year-old woman has consumed over 1 pint of bourbon per day for the past 24 years. She presents with severe cognitive deficits and is diagnosed with Korsakoff syndrome. Which of the following is she most likely to display on mental status examination?

a. Inability to copy a drawn figure
b. Hypermnesia
c. Both anterograde and retrograde memory deficits
d. Retrograde amnesia
e. Retrospective falsification

221. A 55-year-old man comes to the physician with the chief complaint of weight loss and a depressed mood. He feels tired all the time and is no longer interested in the normal activities he previously enjoyed. He feels quite apathetic overall. He has also noticed that he has frequent, nonspecific abdominal pain. Which of the following diagnoses needs to be considered in a patient with this description?

a. Pheochromocytoma
b. Pancreatic carcinoma
c. Adrenocortical insufficiency
d. Cushing syndrome
e. Huntington disease

222. Which of the following is the most common cause of delirium in the elderly?

a. Substance abuse
b. Accidental poisoning
c. Hypoxia
d. Use of multiple medications
e. Alcohol withdrawal

223. A 61-year-old woman comes to the physician with a 6-month history of mild memory loss. She also has had mild-moderate difficulty with calculations which she had previously been able to perform without difficulty. Physical examination and laboratory tests were all within normal limits. Which medication is indicated and should be a first choice for therapy in this case?

a. Tacrine
b. Rivastigmine
c. Galantamine
d. Ondansetron
e. Donepezil

224. A 52-year-old man undergoes a successful mitral valve replacement. He is sent to the intensive care unit to recover. The day after the surgery, he appears irritable and restless. Hours later he is agitated, disoriented, hypervigilant, and uncooperative. This agitation alternates with periods of somnolence. Which of the following is most likely to be helpful?

a. Intramuscular chlorpromazine (Thorazine)
b. Oral alprazolam
c. Modification of environment
d. Oral lithium
e. Supportive psychotherapy

225. A 23-year-old woman comes to the physician with the chief complaint of a depressed mood for 6 months. She states that she has felt lethargic, does not sleep well, and has decreased energy and difficulty concentrating. She notes that she has gained over 15 lb without attempting to do so, and seems to bruise much more easily than previously. On physical examination, she is noted to have numerous purple striae on her abdomen, proximal muscle weakness, and a loss of peripheral vision. A brain tumor is found on MRI. In which of the following areas of the brain was this tumor most likely found?

a. Frontal lobe
b. Cerebellum
c. Thalamus
d. Pituitary
e. Brain stem

226. A 34-year-old man comes to the physician with the chief complaint of new-onset visual hallucinations for 1 month. He states that he sees flashing lights and movement when he knows that there is no one in the room with him. He also complains of a headache that occurs several times per week and is dull and achy in nature. Physical examination reveals papilledema and a homonymous hemianopsia. A brain tumor is found on MRI. In which of the following areas of the brain is this tumor most likely found?

a. Frontal lobe
b. Parietal lobe
c. Occipital lobe
d. Temporal lobe
e. Cerebellum

227. A 26-year-old man comes to the physician with the chief complaint that he has been uncharacteristically moody and irritable. On several occasions his wife has noted that he has had angry outbursts directed at the children and that they were so severe that she had to step in between him and them. He states that he has "spells" in which he smells the odors of rotten eggs and burning rubber. During this time he feels disconnected from his surroundings, as if he were in a dream. A brain tumor is found on MRI. In which of the following areas of the brain is this tumor most likely found?

a. Frontal lobe
b. Parietal lobe
c. Occipital lobe
d. Temporal lobe
e. Cerebellum

228. A 43-year-old man comes to the physician with a 3-month history of nervousness and excitability. He states that he feels this way constantly and that this is a dramatic change for his normally relaxed personality. He notes that on occasion he becomes extremely afraid of his own impending death, even when there is no objective evidence that this would occur. He notes that he has lost 20 lb and frequently has diarrhea. On mental status examination, he is noted to have pressured speech. On physical examination, he is noted to have a fine tremor and tachycardia. Which of the following disorders is this patient most likely to have?

a. Hyperthyroidism
b. Hypothyroidism
c. Hepatic encephalopathy
d. Hyperparathyroidism
e. Hypoparathyroidism

Questions 229 to 233

Match each disorder with the most appropriate test which may be used to either rule the disorder in or rule it out. Each lettered option may be used once, more than once, or not at all.

a. Hematocrit
b. Prolactin
c. Vitamin B_{12}
d. CPK
e. ECG
f. Urine copper
g. Urine vanillylmandelic acid (VMA)
h. Venereal Disease Research Laboratory (VDRL)
i. Serum ammonia

229. Nonepileptic seizures

230. Neuroleptic malignant syndrome

231. Hepatic encephalopathy

232. Tertiary syphilis

233. Pheochromocytoma

234. A 28-year-old woman comes to the physician requesting genetic counseling. Her father has been diagnosed with Huntington disease. What is this woman's risk of developing this disease?

a. 1 in 2.
b. 1 in 4.
c. 1 in 16.
d. 1 in 32.
e. She will not develop the disease, but will be a carrier.

235. A 32-year-old man is admitted to the hospital after he is hit by a car and breaks his femur. Three days into his hospital stay, he tells the nurse that he is repeatedly hearing the voice of his mother telling him to protect himself from danger. He also notes that he sees movement out of the corners of his eyes. He states that these things have never happened to him previously. His vital signs are BP, 160/92 mm/Hg; respirations, 12 breaths/minute; pulse, 110 beats/minute; and temperature, 38°C (100.4°F). Which of the following is the most likely diagnosis for this patient?

a. Delirium tremens
b. Brief psychotic disorder
c. Schizophrenia
d. Schizophreniform disorder
e. Subdural bleed

236. A 42-year-old retired professional boxer is brought to the physician by his wife because his memory is "not what it used to be." She states that she first noticed a small decline in his memory about 15 years after he started boxing (at age 15). However, she notes that his memory has gotten so bad now that she cannot leave him alone in the house. On examination, he is noted to have a moderately severe cognitive impairment. He shows little facial expression and he walks with small, rigid steps. Which of the following is the most likely cause of his disorder?

a. An idiopathic degenerative process
b. Chronic trauma
c. An inborn error of metabolism
d. A familial disorder
e. A vitamin deficiency

237. A 45-year-old woman with no previous psychiatric history is seen in the emergency room for severe agitation, flight of ideas, and delusions of grandeur. The patient states that her only medical problem is rheumatoid arthritis, and although she has been on a number of medications, her rheumatologist prescribed a new one for her recently. Which of the following medications was most likely started by the rheumatologist, precipitating the psychiatric symptoms described in this vignette?

a. Gold
b. Cox 2 inhibitor
c. NSAID
d. Sulfasalazine
e. Corticosteroid

Cognitive Disorders and Consultation-Liaison Psychiatry

Answers

190. The answer is d. (*Jacobson and Jacobson, pp 171-176.*) Alzheimer disease is the most common dementing disorder in North America, Europe, and Scandinavia. Typical symptoms are progressive memory loss, aphasia, anomia (inability to recall the name of objects), apraxia (inability to perform voluntary motor activity but with no motor or sensory deficits), and agnosia (inability to process and understand sensory stimuli but with no sensory deficits). Motor functions are spared until the very end. Personality is preserved in the early stages of the disorder, but considerable deterioration follows in later stages.

191. The answer is b. (*Kaplan and Sadock, pp 341-343.*) Pick disease accounts for 2.5% of cases of dementia. Clinically it is distinguishable from Alzheimer disease by the prominence and early onset of personality changes, disinhibition or apathy, socially inappropriate behavior, mood changes (elation or depression), and psychotic symptoms. Language is affected early in the disease, but the memory loss, apraxia, and agnosia characteristic of Alzheimer disease are not prominent until the late stages of the disorder. Temporofrontal atrophy, demyelination and gliosis of the frontal lobes, Pick bodies (intracellular inclusions), and Pick cells (swollen neurons) are the characteristic pathological findings.

192. The answer is a. (*Kaplan and Sadock, pp 330-335.*) Chronic subdural hematoma causes a reversible form of dementia. It frequently follows head trauma (60% of the cases), with tearing of the bridging veins in the subdural space. Ruptured aneurysms, rapid deceleration injuries, and arterovenous malformations (AVMs) of the pial surface account for the nontraumatic cases. The most common symptoms of chronic subdural hematomas are headache, confusion, inattention, apathy, memory loss, drowsiness, and coma. Lateralization signs, such as hemiparesis, hemianopsia, and cranial nerve abnormalities, are less prominent features. Epidural hematoma usually follows a temporal or parietal skull fracture that causes the laceration of the middle meningeal artery or vein. It is characterized by a brief period of lucidity followed by loss of consciousness, hemiparesis, cranial nerve palsies, and death, unless the hematoma is surgically evacuated. Multi-infarct dementia and Alzheimer disease are characterized by a slower onset and have a more chronic course, although diagnostic confusion is possible at times. Korsakoff disorder is characterized by anterograde and retrograde memory deficits. Frontal lobe tumors mainly present with personality and behavioral changes, which vary depending on the localization.

193. The answer is a. *(Kaplan and Sadock, pp 639-641.)* A conversion disorder usually presents in a monosymptomatic manner, acutely, and simulating a physical disease. The sensory or motor symptoms present are not fully explained by any known pathophysiology. The diagnostic features are such that the physical symptom is incompatible with known physiological mechanisms or anatomy. Usually an unconscious psychological stress or conflict is present. In hypochondriasis, a patient is overly concerned that he or she has an illness or illnesses; this conviction can temporarily be appeased by physician reassurance, but the reassurance generally does not last long. Factitious disorder usually presents with physical or mental symptoms that are induced by the patient to meet the psychological need to be taken care of (primary gain). Malingering is similar to factitious disorder in that symptoms are faked, but the motive in malingering is some secondary gain, such as getting out of jail. In delusional disorder with somatic delusions, the patient has an unshakable belief that he or she has some physical defect or a medical condition.

194. The answer is b. *(Kaplan and Sadock, pp 325, 327.)* This patient presents with a rather classic picture of a substance-induced delirium. In this case, an elderly person was started on a benzodiazepine for sleep. Benzodiazepines in the elderly must be used with extreme caution, if at all, because of their potential for delirium or a paradoxical excitation effect. The incoherence, waxing and waning of consciousness, and psychotic symptoms (hypervigilance, paranoia, and disorganized thoughts) also point to a delirium.

195. The answer is e. *(Moore and Jefferson, pp 308-311.)* In partial complex seizures, an altered state of consciousness, usually manifested by staring, is accompanied by hallucinations (olfactory hallucinations are common), automatisms (buttoning and unbuttoning, masticatory movements, speech automatisms), perceptual alterations (objects changing shape or size), complex verbalizations, and autonomic symptoms such as piloerection, gastric sensation, or nausea. Flashbacks, déjà vu, and derealization are also common. The episodes last approximately 1 minute and patients may experience postictal headaches and sleepiness. Absence seizure episodes are shorter, are not accompanied by motor activity, and are not followed by postictal phenomena.

196. The answer is a. (*Moore and Jefferson, pp 221-223.*) Sleep apnea is the cessation of breathing during sleep for 10 seconds or more. In obstructive sleep apnea, breathing stops owing to airway blockage, while in central sleep apnea, the breathing stops because of an absence of respiratory efforts secondary to a neurological dysfunction. Features associated with obstructive sleep apnea are excessive daytime somnolence, snoring, restless sleep, and nocturnal awakening with gasping for air. Patients often wake up in the morning with dry mouth and headache. Predisposing factors are maleness, middle age, obesity, hypothyroidism, and various malformations of the upper airways. Narcolepsy is characterized by irresistible urges to fall asleep for brief periods during the day, regardless of the situation. Nocturnal myoclonus refers to stereotyped, repetitive movements of the legs during sleep, accompanied by brief arousal and sleep disruption.

197. The answer is c. (*Kaplan and Sadock, pp 792-794.*) Patients with borderline personalities see others (and themselves) as wholly good or totally bad, a psychological defense called *splitting*. They alternatively idealize or devalue important figures in their lives, depending on their perceptions of the others' intentions, interest, and level of caring. These dynamics often elicit similar responses in the environment, with the individuals being idealized having a considerably better opinion of the patient than those who are being devalued.

198. The answer is c. (*Kaplan and Sadock, p 368.*) Cushing syndrome caused by exogenous administration of corticosteroids, and more rarely to adrenocarcinoma or ectopic production of ACTH, is often associated with psychiatric disturbances. Depression and mixed anxiety and depressive states are the most common psychiatric manifestations of the syndrome (from 35% to 68%, depending on the study). Since the affective symptoms are directly secondary to the administration of a substance (in this case, steroids for the treatment of asthma), the patient's diagnosis would be a substance-induced mood disorder. Mania, psychosis, delirium, and cognitive disturbances also occur, but at a much lower rate. Depressive symptoms occur early in the disorder (in the prodromal period in 27% of cases). Most patients improve after the primary disorder is treated and serum cortisol decreases.

199. The answer is a. *(Kaplan and Sadock, p 328.)* Haloperidol is a commonly used drug to treat the psychotic symptoms that may be apparent in delirious patients. If the patient is agitated, the drug can be safely given IM, but should be switched over to a low dose of oral medication as soon as the patient is willing and/or able to do so. Drugs with significant anticholinergic activity should be avoided in delirious patients, as should benzodiazepines in the elderly.

200. The answer is c. *(Kaplan and Sadock, p 333.)* Huntington disease is a neurodegenerative disorder characterized by choreic movements of the face, limbs, and trunk; progressive dementia; and psychiatric symptoms. Deficits in sustained attention, memory retrieval, procedural memory (ability to acquire new skills), and visuospatial skills are predominant and early manifestations of the disorder. Language skills are usually preserved until the late stages of the disease. Personality changes and mood disturbances, including depression and mania, are frequent and can predate the onset of the dementia and the movement disorder. Neuroimaging reveals atrophy of the caudate and the putamen.

201. The answer is c. *(Kaplan and Sadock, p 1142.)* Impaired naming, memory deterioration, poor calculation, poor judgment, and disinhibition are characteristic symptoms of Alzheimer disease. Neurofibrillary tangles, neuritic plaques, and loss of acetylcholine neurons in the nucleus basalis of Meynert—pathological changes characteristic of Alzheimer disease—develop in patients with Down syndrome at a relatively young adult age. Estimates suggest that 25% or more of individuals with Down syndrome over age 35 show the signs and symptoms of Alzheimer-type dementia. The percentage increases with age. The incidence of Alzheimer disease in people with Down syndrome is estimated to be three to five times greater than that of the general population. Current research shows that the extra "gene dosage" caused by the abnormal third chromosome of Down syndrome may be a factor in the development of Alzheimer disease. The early aging of the Down syndrome brain may also be a factor.

202. The answer is a. *(Kaplan and Sadock, pp 341-343.)* Multi-infarct dementia results from the cumulative effects of multiple small- and large-vessel occlusions in cortical and subcortical regions. Most cases are caused by hypertensive cerebrovascular disease and thrombo-occlusive disease. It is the second most common cause of dementia in the elderly, accounting for 8% to 35% of the cases. Clinically, it is characterized by memory and cognitive deficits accompanied by focal neurologic signs (muscle weakness, spasticity, dysarthria, extensor plantar reflex, etc). Unlike Alzheimer disease, multi-infarct dementia is characterized by sudden onset and a stepwise progression.

203. The answer is c. *(Moore and Jefferson, pp 421-422.)* Creutzfeldt-Jakob disease is a neurodegenerative disease caused by a transmissible infectious agent, the prion. Most cases are iatrogenic, following transplant of infected corneas or use of contaminated neurosurgical instruments. Familial forms, following an autosomal dominant pattern of inheritance, represent 5% to 15% of cases. Patients show a very rapid cognitive deterioration, myoclonic jerks, rigidity, and ataxia. Death follows within a year. An intermittent periodic burst pattern (periodic complexes) is the characteristic EEG finding. Epilepsy causes spike and wave patterns on EEG, and may cause postseizure memory loss and disorientation (in generalized, tonic-clonic seizures) or a depersonalization syndrome (in temporal lobe epilepsy or other focal seizure disorder), but would not be expected to cause dementia, continuous myoclonic jerks on examination, or an EEG that shows periodic bursts of electrical activity superimposed on a slow background. *Pseudodementia* is the term used for patients with major depression, who exhibit impaired attention, perception, problem solving, or memory. The cognitive decline is often more precipitous than for demented patients. Patient history often reveals past major depressive episodes. Although the actual memory impairment is modest in these patients, the subjective complaint is great.

204. The answer is c. *(Moore and Jefferson, pp 257-258.)* This patient is demonstrating some very characteristic signs and symptoms of a person with a narcissistic personality disorder. His wife states that this kind of behavior is not new for this patient, making any of the more acute disorders unlikely. Patients with narcissistic personality disorder, in the face of some narcissistic insult (in this case, the myocardial infarction, reminding the patient that he is, indeed just human), often react with an exaggerated denial of the problem. In this case, the patient jumps down and does push-ups, to "prove" he has not been affected by the myocardial infarction. Approaches to this patient that do not involve direct confrontation but, rather, work with the patient's need to be admired are more likely to be successful.

205. The answer is c. (*Kaplan and Sadock, pp 591-593.*) Hyperventilation causes hypocapnia and respiratory alkalosis, which in turn lead to decreased cerebral blood flow and a decrease in ionized serum calcium. Dizziness, derealization, and light-headedness are caused by the cerebral vasoconstriction, while circumoral tingling, carpopedal spasm, and paresthesias are symptoms of hypocalcemia. Hyperventilation is a central feature of panic disorder and acute anxiety attacks, though more symptoms are required (beyond just hyperventilation) to make those diagnoses. Panic disorder is characterized by recurring, spontaneous, and unexpected anxiety attacks with rapid onset and short duration. The symptoms of an attack climb to maximum intensity within 10 minutes, but can peak within a few seconds. Typical symptoms include shortness of breath, tachypnea, tachycardia, tremor, dizziness, hot or cold sensations, chest discomfort, and feelings of depersonalization or derealization. A minimum of four symptoms is required to meet the diagnosis of panic attack. Generalized anxiety disorder is characterized by excessive anxiety and worry, occurring more days than not for at least 6 months, about a number of events or activities. The anxiety and worry are associated with three or more of six symptoms: (1) restlessness or feeling keyed up or on edge, (2) becoming easily fatigued, (3) difficulty concentrating, (4) irritability, (5) muscle tension, and (6) sleep disturbance. Anxiety disorder not otherwise specified is characterized by similar constellations of symptoms with one of the other *Diagnostic and Statistical Manual, 4th edition* (*DSM-IV*) diagnoses (panic disorder, phobia, GAD, PTSD [posttraumatic stress disorder], etc). There are insufficient criteria to meet any one of the diagnoses, but perhaps a number of symptoms for several. Anxiety disorder secondary to a general medical condition is characterized by symptoms of anxiety, but these symptoms must be related to (and caused by) a medical illness, such as hyperthyroidism, angina, hypoglycemia, and so on.

206. The answer is c. (*Kaplan and Sadock, p 819.*) Given that the diagnosis in this case is hyperventilation, the treatment of choice is rebreathing into a paper bag. In doing so, the hypocapnia is reversed, as is the respiratory alkalosis, which in turn leads to a return of normal cerebral blood flow and a normalization of the ionized serum calcium. All signs and symptoms will disappear from there. After the hyperventilation episodes are stopped, it might be advisable for the patient to learn relaxation techniques (perhaps through biofeedback or hypnosis) so that the episodes will not recur. Neither a benzodiazepine nor an antidepressant is indicated in this case.

207. The answer is b. (*Kaplan and Sadock, p 89.*) Temporal lobe epilepsy (TLE) may often manifest as bizarre behavior without the classic grand mal shaking movements caused by seizures in the motor cortex. A TLE personality is characterized by hyposexuality, emotional intensity, and a perseverative approach to interactions, termed *viscosity*. Wernicke-Korsakoff syndrome is a neurologic condition manifested by confusion, ataxia, and nystagmus; thiamine deficiency is its direct cause. If thiamine is given during the acute stage of Wernicke encephalopathy, Korsakoff syndrome can be prevented. This syndrome is characterized by a severe anterograde learning defect associated with confabulations. Although Wernicke-Korsakoff can be caused by malnutrition alone, it is usually associated with alcohol abuse and dependence. Pick disease is a form of frontal lobe dementia in which Pick cells and bodies (irregularly shaped, silver-staining, intracytoplasmic inclusion bodies that displace the nucleus toward the periphery) are present in the brain. There is an insidious onset and gradual progression, with early decline in social interpersonal conduct. Emotional blunting and apathy also occur early without insight into them. There is a marked decline in personal hygiene and significant distractibility and motor impersistence.

208. The answer is c. (*Kaplan and Sadock, p 334.*) HIV dementia is the most frequent neurological complication of HIV infection and can be the first symptom of the infection. It is caused by a direct effect of the virus on the brain and is always accompanied by some brain atrophy. HIV dementia presents with the combination of cognitive impairment, motor deficits, and behavioral changes typical of a subcortical dementia. Common features include impaired attention and concentration, psychomotor slowing, forgetfulness, slow reaction time, and mood changes.

209 and 210. The answers are 209-d, 210-e. (*Kaplan and Sadock, p 844.*) Wernicke encephalopathy occurs in nutritionally deficient alcoholics and is because of thiamine deficiency and consequent damage of the thiamine-dependent brain structures, including the mammillary bodies and the dorsomedial nucleus of the thalamus. It presents with mental confusion, ataxia, and sixth-nerve paralysis. Wernicke encephalopathy is a medical emergency and can rapidly resolve with immediate supplementation of thiamine. This diagnosis should be considered in any patient brought into the emergency room unresponsive.

211. The answer is e. (*Moore and Jefferson, pp 384-385.*) Normal-pressure hydrocephalus (NPH) is an idiopathic disorder caused by the obstruction of the flow of the cerebrospinal fluid into the subarachnoid space. Onset usually occurs after age 60. The classic syndrome of NPH consists of urinary incontinence, gait abnormality, and dementia (wet, wobbly, and wacky). The dementia displays frontal-subcortical dysfunction features, such as impaired attention, visuospatial deficits, and poor judgment. Apathy, inertia, and lack of concern are the typical personality changes. Ventricular dilatation without sulcal widening (ie, without evidence of atrophy) and normal CSF pressure during lumbar puncture are diagnostic. The dementia can be reversed with a CSF shunt, especially if the course of the disease is short. Careful history will likely reveal the progression of symptoms as first gait, followed by incontinence, followed by dementia in NPH. The absence of involuntary movements in this patient make Parkinson disease less likely than NPH.

212 to 214. The answers are 212-d, 213-a, 214-b. (*Jacobson and Jacobson, pp 153, 157, 159.*) Factitious disorder usually presents with physical or mental symptoms that are induced by the patient to meet the psychological need to be taken care of (primary gain). These patients will often mutilate themselves repeatedly in a frantic effort to be cared for by the hospital system. Moving between hospitals so that they don't get caught is common, especially when the patient is directly confronted. Malingering is similar to factitious disorder in that symptoms are faked, but the motive for malingering is some secondary gain, such as getting out of jail. Somatization disorder is characterized by the recurrent physical complaints that are not explained by physical factors and that cause significant impairment or result in seeking medical attention. Pain of any part of the body and dysfunctions of multiple systems are typical. The *DSM-IV* diagnostic criteria for somatization disorder include at least four pain symptoms, one sexual symptom, and one pseudoneurological symptom. These symptoms can be present at any time in the duration of the disorder. Somatization disorder usually emerges in adolescence or the early twenties and follows a chronic course. Somatization disorder is diagnosed predominantly in women, with a prevalence of 0.2% to 0.5%, and rarely in men. Body dysmorphic disorder is characterized by distorted beliefs about the patient's own appearance, often with delusional qualities. Borderline personality disorder patients may mutilate themselves, but the object is generally to get attention or relieve stress.

215. The answer is d. (*Kaplan and Sadock, p 491.*) Neuroleptic medications can produce hyperprolactinemia even at very low doses and are the most common cause of galactorrhea in psychiatric patients. Hyperprolactinemia with neuroleptic use is secondary to the blockade of dopamine receptors with these drugs. (Dopamine normally inhibits prolactin, and with dopamine's blockade, hyperprolactinemia can result.) Amenorrhea and galactorrhea are the main symptoms of hyperprolactinemia in women, and impotence is the main symptom in men, although men can also develop gynecomastia and galactorrhea. Other causes of hyperprolactinemia include severe systemic illness such as cirrhosis or renal failure, pituitary tumors, idiopathic sources, and pregnancy.

216. The answer is c. (*Kaplan and Sadock, p 372.*) Acute arsenic poisoning from ingestion results in increased permeability of small blood vessels and inflammation and necrosis of the intestinal mucosa; these changes manifest as hemorrhagic gastroenteritis, fluid loss, and hypotension. Symptoms include nausea, vomiting, diarrhea, abdominal pain, delirium, coma, and seizures. A garlicky odor may be detectable on the breath. Arsenic is found in herbal and homeopathic remedies, insecticides, rodenticides, and wood preservatives, and it has a variety of other industrial applications.

217. The answer is d. (*Jacobson and Jacobson, pp 154-156.*) Hypochondriasis is recognized by the patient's preoccupation with having a serious medical condition based on the misinterpretation of his or her own bodily symptoms. Despite medical evaluation and reassurance, the patient continues to fear that the disease is present. Often, after reassurance is given (usually because a negative test result is received) the patient is temporarily relieved, but this relief does not last. The symptoms must cause clinically significant distress, and be present for longer than 6 months.

218. The answer is c. (*Jacobson and Jacobson, pp 154-156.*) The patient should be referred to a primary care doctor who will see her regularly but not perform any invasive procedures unless there is a clear indication to do so. New complaints or fears about an illness should be dealt with by the primary care physician, using a limited evaluation (history or physical examination) to ensure that no organic disease has developed, since even patients with hypochondriasis can become physically ill. Since these patients do not believe that their disorder is psychiatric, referral for psychotherapy is likely to be unsuccessful. The patient in this question reports no other signs of depression, and thus an antidepressant is not warranted. Likewise, though she has a recurrent complaint/concern about ovarian cancer, this does not rise to delusional proportions—she is capable of being reassured, at least for a time, by negative results. Presuming the patient has already had a work-up for ovarian cancer, which it appears by history that she has, further work-up for this disease is unwarranted.

219. The answer is d. *(Kaplan and Sadock, p 991.)* A placebo is an inactive substance disguised as an active treatment. It can be effective in treating pain with both psychogenic and organic causes. Consequently, the only conclusion that can be reached about the man described in the question is that he responds to placebos. His response says nothing about whether his pain is real or psychogenic. Many psychological factors are thought to contribute to the effects of placebos, including the patient's expectations, the provider's attitude toward the patient and the treatment, and conditioned responses.

220. The answer is c. *(Kaplan and Sadock, p 338.)* Korsakoff psychosis is characterized by both anterograde and retrograde memory deficits. Patients cannot form new memories, and they have difficulties recalling past personal events, with the poorest recall for events that took place closest to the onset of the amnesia. Remote memories are usually preserved. Using the mnemonic RACK may help students remember the characteristics of Korsakoff psychosis: Retrograde and anterograde amnesia; Confabulation; Korsakoff syndrome.

221. The answer is b. *(Kaplan and Sadock, pp 830-832.)* Pancreatic carcinoma should always be considered in depressed middle-aged patients. It presents with weight loss, abdominal pain, apathy, decreased energy, lethargy, anhedonia, and depression. An elevated amylase can sometimes be found in laboratory testing. The other disorders listed do not present in this manner.

222. The answer is d. *(Jacobson and Jacobson, pp 177-181.)* The use of multiple medications (polypharmacy) is among the most common causes of delirium in elderly patients, especially patients who already show signs of cognitive deterioration and many medical problems. Drug abuse and drug withdrawal are more commonly seen in young and middle-aged adults. Accidental poisoning and hypoxia (eg, from drowning) are more frequent in children.

223. The answer is e. (*Kaplan and Sadock, p 343.*) Donepezil, rivastigmine, galantamine, and tacrine are cholinesterase inhibitors that can all be used to treat the mild to moderate symptoms of Alzheimer dementia. However, as a first-choice therapy, donepezil should be chosen as it is well tolerated. Tacrine has a potential for hepatotoxicity which makes it a less favorable first choice. Revastigmine and galantamine are more likely to cause gastrointestinal distress and/or neuropsychiatric side effects, which also makes it a less favorable first choice. Ondansetron is still under investigation, so it would not be a first choice therapy in this patient.

224. The answer is c. (*Kaplan and Sadock, p 324.*) Postcardiotomy delirium is a frequent complication of cardiac surgery, with a prevalence that has remained constant through the years at 32%. Among the identified causes of this syndrome have been drug effects, especially from opioids and anticholinergic medications; subclinical brain injury; complement activation; poor nutritional status; and embolism. Stable vital signs help in the differential diagnosis with delirium tremens, which is accompanied by hypertension, tachycardia, and elevated temperature. The addition of medications to this picture usually does not help, and may worsen the condition. If medication is necessary to control agitation, a small dose of a *high-potency* neuroleptic is the treatment of choice. (The use of intramuscular thorazine, a low-potency neuroleptic presented as option "a" in this question, would therefore be a bad choice regardless.) Frequent orientation of the patient to his or her surroundings by facility personnel usually helps. Other modifications of the environment that might prove helpful include putting a clock or calendar in the room and bringing familiar items from home.

225. The answer is d. (*Kaplan and Sadock, p 821.*) Tumors of the pituitary cause bitemporal hemianopsia by compressing the optic chiasm and a variety of endocrine disturbances that in turn can cause psychiatric symptoms. The woman in the question has a basophilic adenoma, and her depression is part of her Cushing syndrome. Patients with craniopharyngiomas can also present with behavioral and autonomic disturbances caused by the upward extension of the tumor into the diencephalon.

226. The answer is c. *(Kaplan and Sadock, pp 74-75.)* Occipital lobe tumors present with headache, papilledema, and homonymous hemianopsia. Visual problems and seizures are common. Patients may also complain of visual hallucinations or auras of flashing lights and movement.

227. The answer is d. *(Kaplan and Sadock, pp 76-77.)* Tumors of the temporal lobe can present with olfactory and other unusual types of hallucinations, derealization episodes, mood lability, irritability, intermittent anger, and behavioral dyscontrol. Anxiety is another frequent finding.

228. The answer is a. *(Kaplan and Sadock, p 820.)* Patients with hyperthyroidism complain of heat intolerance and excessive sweating, as well as diarrhea, weight loss, tachycardia, palpitations, and vomiting. Psychiatric complaints can include nervousness, excitability, irritability, pressured speech, insomnia, psychosis, and a fear of impending death or doom. Decreased concentration, hyperactivity, and a fine tremor may also be found.

229 to 233. The answers are 229-b, 230-d, 231-i, 232-h, 233-g. *(Kaplan and Sadock, pp 262-266.)* Grand mal seizures are followed by a sharp rise in serum prolactin level that lasts approximately 20 minutes. Since in nonepileptic seizures prolactin levels do not change, this test may be helpful in the differential diagnosis to rule out epileptic seizures, leaving the diagnosis of nonepileptic seizures as much more likely. In neuroleptic malignant syndrome, the severe muscle contraction causes rhabdomyolysis and an increase of the serum CPK level. CPK levels also increase with dystonic reactions and following intramuscular injections. Serum ammonia is increased in delirium secondary to hepatic encephalopathy. Gastrointestinal hemorrhages and severe cardiac failure may also cause an increase in serum ammonia. A VDRL is helpful in the diagnosis of tertiary syphilis, which can present with irresponsible behavior, irritability, and confusion. A pheochromocytoma, diagnosed with a urine VMA, may present with a variety of psychiatric symptoms, including anxiety, apprehension, panic, diaphoresis, and tremor.

234. The answer is a. *(Moore and Jefferson, pp 326-328.)* Huntington disease is an autosomal dominant disorder, and in affected families the risk for developing the disease is 50%. Huntington disease has been traced to an area of unstable DNA on chromosome 4.

235. The answer is a. (*Kaplan and Sadock, p 829.*) The most common cause of new-onset hallucinations in a recently hospitalized patient is delirium tremens. The onset in this question (3 days) is classic—3 to 4 days after hospitalization is the norm for this disorder to appear, since that is the normal time course for withdrawal symptoms from alcohol to appear. The clues to this diagnosis lie in the facts that the patient has not had these symptoms before (the sudden onset of schizophrenia or schizophreniform disorder in a 34-year-old man with no previous history of psychosis is unlikely) and that he has elevated vital signs. While it is conceivable that this patient could have a brief psychotic disorder, it is much less likely than delirium tremens, given the history and the patient's vital signs. Subdural bleeds would likewise not affect vital signs, and other symptoms, such as disorientation, altered level of consciousness, or a headache, would likely be present.

236. The answer is b. (*Kaplan and Sadock, p 334.*) A persisting dementia called chronic traumatic encephalopathy occurs with multiple head traumas, even of minor entity. A classic example is dementia pugilistica, or boxer's dementia. In this disorder, cognitive decline and memory deficits are characteristically accompanied by parkinsonian symptoms.

237. The answer is e. (*Kaplan and Sadock, p 460.*) Corticosteroids are notorious for precipitating mood changes in patients begun on them. A common mood change is that of hypomania or mania, which often changes to a depressed mood with chronic administration of the steroid. Steroid withdrawal may also cause both manic and depressive mood features.

Schizophrenia and Other Psychotic Disorders

Questions

238. A 24-year-old man with chronic schizophrenia is brought to the emergency room after his parents found him in his bed and were unable to communicate with him. On examination, the man is confused and disoriented. He has severe muscle rigidity and a temperature of 39.4°C (103°F). His blood pressure is elevated, and he has a leucocytosis. Which of the following is the best first step in the pharmacologic treatment of this man?

a. Haloperidol
b. Lorazepam
c. Bromocriptine
d. Benztropine
e. Lithium

239. A 54-year-old man with a chronic mental illness seems to be constantly chewing. He does not wear dentures. His tongue darts in and out of his mouth, and he occasionally smacks his lips. He also grimaces, frowns, and blinks excessively. Which of the following disorders is most likely in this patient?

a. Tourette syndrome
b. Akathisia
c. Tardive dyskinesia
d. Parkinson disease
e. Huntington disease

240. A 58-year-old woman with a chronic mental disorder comes to the physician with irregular choreoathetoid movements of her hands and trunk. She states that the movements get worse under stressful conditions. Which of the following medications is most likely to have caused this disorder?

a. Fluoxetine
b. Clozapine
c. Perphenazine
d. Diazepam
e. Phenobarbitol

241. A 19-year-old woman is brought to the emergency room by her roommate after the patient told her that, "the voices are telling me to kill the teacher." The roommate states the patient has always been isolative and "odd" but for the past 2 weeks she has been hoarding food, talking to herself, and appearing very paranoid. Which of the following features would be indicative of a good prognosis with respect to this disease?

a. Young onset
b. Withdrawn behavior
c. Poor support system
d. Family history of mood disorders
e. Neurologic signs and symptoms present

242. The patient in question 241 becomes very agitated in the emergency room, screaming that the nurses were there to kill her and that she had to escape. She tried to strike one of the nurses before being restrained. Which of the following treatment options is recommended first?

a. Haloperidol and lorazepam IM
b. Clozapine PO
c. Fluphenazine decanoate IM
d. Thioridazine (Mellaril) IM
e. Lorazepam PO

243. The patient in the above vignette was admitted and started on a daily dose of fluphenazine. After discharge from the hospital, she was kept on a low dose of the medication for 6 weeks. She showed only a minimal response to the drug, even after it was raised to a moderate dosage level. Which of the following is the next therapeutic step?

a. Give a high dose of fluphenazine.
b. Give a low dose of clozaril.
c. Give a low dose of haloperidol.
d. Give fluphenazine decanoate IM.
e. Give a low dose of olanzapine.

244. A 24-year-old woman comes to the emergency room with the chief complaint that "my stomach is rotting out from the inside." She states that for the last 6 months she has been crying on a daily basis and that she has decreased concentration, energy, and interest in her usual hobbies. She has lost 25 lb during that time. She cannot get to sleep, and when she does, she wakes up early in the morning. For the past 3 weeks, she has become convinced that she is dying of cancer and is rotting on the inside of her body. Also, in the past 2 weeks she has been hearing a voice calling her name when no one is around. Which of the following is the most likely diagnosis?

a. Delusional disorder
b. Schizoaffective disorder
c. Schizophreniform disorder
d. Schizophrenia
e. Major depression with psychotic features

245. A 19-year-old man is brought to the physician by his parents after he called them from college, terrified that the Mafia was after him. He reports that he has eaten nothing for the past 6 weeks other than canned beans because "they are into everything—I can't be too careful." He is convinced that the Mafia has put cameras in his dormitory room and that they are watching his every move. He occasionally hears the voices of two men talking about him when no one is around. His roommate states that for the past 2 months the patient has been increasingly withdrawn and suspicious. Which of the following is the most likely diagnosis?

a. Delusional disorder
b. Schizoaffective disorder
c. Schizophreniform disorder
d. Schizophrenia
e. Phencyclidine (PCP) intoxication

246. A 36-year-old woman is brought to the psychiatrist by her husband because for the past 8 months she has refused to go out of the house, believing that the neighbors are trying to harm her. She is afraid that if they see her they will hurt her, and she finds many small bits of evidence to support this. This evidence includes the neighbors' leaving their garbage cans out on the street to try to trip her, parking their cars in their driveways so they can hide behind them and spy on her, and walking by her house to try to get a look into where she is hiding. She states that her mood is fine and would be "better if they would leave me alone." She denies hearing the neighbors or anyone else talk to her, but is sure that they are out to "cause her death and mayhem." Which of the following is the most likely diagnosis?

a. Delusional disorder
b. Schizophreniform disorder
c. Schizoaffective disorder
d. Schizophrenia
e. Major depression with psychotic features

247. A 35-year-old woman has lived in a state psychiatric hospital for the past 10 years. She spends most of her day rocking, muttering softly to herself, or looking at her reflection in a small mirror. She needs help with dressing and showering, and she often giggles and laughs for no apparent reason. Which of the following is the most likely diagnosis?

a. Schizophrenia
b. Delusional disorder
c. Bipolar disorder, manic phase
d. Schizoaffective disorder
e. Schizophreniform disorder

248. A 20-year-old woman is brought to the emergency room by her family because they have been unable to get her to eat or drink anything for the past 2 days. The patient, although awake, is completely unresponsive both vocally and nonverbally. She actively resists any attempt to be moved. Her family reports that during the previous 7 months she became increasingly withdrawn, socially isolated, and bizarre; often speaking to people no one else could see. Which of the following is the most likely diagnosis?

a. Schizoaffective disorder
b. Delusional disorder
c. Schizophreniform disorder
d. Catatonia
e. PCP intoxication

249. A 21-year-old man is brought to the emergency room by his parents because he has not slept, bathed, or eaten in the past 3 days. The parents report that for the past 6 months their son has been acting strangely and "not himself." They state that he has been locking himself in his room, talking to himself, and writing on the walls. Six weeks prior to the emergency room visit, their son became convinced that a fellow student was stealing his thoughts and making him unable to learn his school material. In the past 2 weeks, they have noticed that their son has become depressed and has stopped taking care of himself, including bathing, eating, and getting dressed. On examination, the patient is dirty, disheveled, and crying. He complains of not being able to concentrate, a low energy level, and feeling suicidal. Which of the following is the most likely diagnosis for this patient?

a. Schizoaffective disorder
b. Schizophrenia
c. Bipolar I disorder
d. Schizoid personality disorder
e. Delusional disorder

250. A 47-year-old woman is brought to the emergency room after she jumped off an overpass in a suicide attempt. In the emergency room she states that she wanted to kill herself because the devil had been tormenting her for many years. Her mood is observed to be dysphoric, and she has symptoms of anhedonia, decreased concentration, and anergia. After stabilization of her fractures, she is admitted to the psychiatric unit, where she is treated with risperidone and sertraline. After 2 weeks she is no longer suicidal and her mood is euthymic. However, she still believes that the devil is recruiting people to try to persecute her. In the past 10 years, the patient has had three similar episodes prior to this one. Throughout this time, she has never stopped believing that the devil is persecuting her. Which of the following is the most appropriate diagnosis for this patient?

a. Delusional disorder
b. Schizoaffective disorder
c. Schizophrenia, paranoid type
d. Schizophreniform disorder
e. Major depression with psychotic features

251. A 40-year-old woman is arrested by the police after she is found crawling through the window of a movie star's home. She states that the movie star invited her into his home because the two are secretly married and "it just wouldn't be good for his career if everyone knew." The movie star denies the two have ever met, but notes that the woman has sent him hundreds of letters over the past 2 years. The woman has never been in trouble before and lives an otherwise isolated and unremarkable life. Which of the following is the most likely diagnosis?

a. Delusional disorder
b. Schizoaffective disorder
c. Bipolar I disorder
d. Cyclothymia
e. Schizophreniform disorder

Questions 252 to 256

Match each type of delusional disorder with the vignette which best describes it. Each lettered option may be used once, more than once, or not at all.

a. Erotomanic
b. Grandiose
c. Jealous
d. Persecutory
e. Somatic
f. Mixed
g. Unspecified

252. A 48-year-old woman becomes convinced that her next-door neighbor hates her and wants her to move. She states she has evidence, and when asked to explain, tells the psychiatrist that the neighbor gives her "looks," puts excessive junk in her mailbox, and leaves yard clippings on her side of the yard to harass her.

253. A 62-year-old man is arrested for disturbing people on their way to work by insisting they take his prepared reading materials with them. The topic of the materials was the man's special communications with God and his instructions for following him on a special path to heaven.

254. A 49-year-old man was arrested for beating up on his wife. He stated he had to punish her for having an affair—which she vehemently denied. The man's wife states to the police that the man has accused her of being interested in many other men over the course of their marriage. He now seems fixated on the topic.

255. A 19-year-old college student came to his primary care doctor for help with a foul odor he believed he was unintentionally emitting. The student stated that the odor left him socially isolated and that he was miserable about it. The primary care doctor could detect no odor.

256. A 58-year-old man called the police on his neighbors because he felt they were against him. When asked why, the man explained that the neighbors knew that he was a genius inventor, and they were unhappy about this because his impending fame would disrupt the neighborhood.

257. A 30-year-old man is brought to the emergency room after he was found wandering on the streets with no shoes in the middle of winter. He is admitted to the inpatient psychiatric unit and stabilized on antipsychotic medication. Looking at past records, his psychiatrist notes that he is repeatedly noncompliant with his medication postdischarge, and each time he relapses within 6 months. Which of the following medications is the best one on which to maintain this patient?

a. Clozapine
b. Haloperidol decanoate
c. Chlorpromazine
d. Thioridazine
e. Quetiapine

258. A 26-year-old woman is brought to the emergency room by her husband after she begins screaming that her children are calling to her and becomes hysterical. The husband states that 2 weeks previously, the couple's two children were killed in a car accident, and since that time the patient has been agitated, disorganized, and incoherent. He states that she will not eat because she believes he has been poisoning her food, and she has not slept for the past 2 days. The patient believes that the nurses in the emergency room are going to cause her harm as well. The patient is sedated and later sent home. One week later, all her symptoms remit spontaneously. Which of the following is the most likely diagnosis for this patient?

a. Delirium
b. Schizophreniform disorder
c. Major depression with psychotic features
d. Brief psychotic disorder
e. Posttraumatic stress disorder

259. A 28-year-old woman is brought to see a psychiatrist by her mother. The patient insists that nothing is wrong with her, but the mother notes that the patient has been slowly but progressively isolating herself from everyone. She now rarely leaves the house. The mother says she can hear the patient talking to "people who aren't there" while she's in her room. On examination, the patient is noted to have auditory hallucinations and the delusional belief that her mother is going to kick her out of the house so that it can be turned into a theme park. Which of the following is the lifetime prevalence for this disorder?

a. 1%
b. 3%
c. 5%
d. 10%
e. 15%

260. A 25-year-old woman is diagnosed with schizophrenia when, after the sudden death of her mother, she begins complaining about hearing the voice of the devil and is suddenly afraid that other people are out to hurt her. Her history indicates that she has also experienced a 3-year period of slowly worsening social withdrawal, apathy, and bizarre behavior. Her family history includes major depression in her father. Which of the following details of her history leads the physician to suspect that her outcome may be poor?

a. She is female.
b. She was age 25 at diagnosis.
c. She had an acute precipitating factor before she began hearing voices.
d. She had an insidious onset of her illness.
e. There is a history of affective disorder in her family.

261. A 22-year-old man is brought to the emergency room after he became exceedingly anxious in his college dormitory room, stating that he was sure the college administration was sending a "hit squad" to kill him. He also notes that he can see "visions" of men dressed in black who are carrying guns and stalking him. His thought process is relatively intact, without thought blocking or loose associations. His urine toxicology screen is positive for one of the following drugs. Which drug is the most likely cause of these symptoms?

a. Barbiturates
b. Heroin
c. Benzodiazepines
d. Amphetamines
e. MDMA (Ecstasy)

262. A 72-year-old woman is brought to the emergency room by her daughter after she found her mother rummaging in the garbage cans outside her home. The daughter states that the patient has never had any behavior like this previously. On interview, the patient states she sees "martians hiding around her home, and on occasion, hears them too." She also demonstrates a constructional apraxia, with difficulty drawing a clock and intersecting pentagons. All except one of these symptoms point to a medical cause for this patient's behavior. Which symptom is most common in a purely psychiatric disorder?

a. Patient's age
b. No previous history of this behavior
c. Visual hallucinations
d. Auditory hallucinations
e. Constructional apraxia

263. Families of patients with schizophrenia, who are overtly hostile and overly controlling, affect the patient in which one of the following ways?

a. Increased relapse rate
b. Decreased rate of compliance
c. High likelihood that this behavior led to the patient's first break of the disease
d. Increased likelihood that the patient's schizophrenia will be of the paranoid type
e. Decreased risk of suicidal behavior

264. A 62-year-old man with chronic schizophrenia is brought to the emergency room after he is found wandering around his halfway house, confused and disoriented. His serum sodium concentration is 123 meq/L and urine sodium concentration is 5 meq/L. The patient has been treated with risperidone 4 mg/day for the past 3 years with good symptom control. His roommate reports that the patient often complains of feeling thirsty. Which of the following is the most likely cause of this patient's symptoms?

a. Renal failure
b. Inappropriate antidiuretic hormone (ADH) secretion
c. Addison disease
d. Psychogenic polydipsia
e. Nephrotic syndrome

265. A 23-year-old woman was diagnosed with schizophrenia after a single episode of psychosis (hallucinations and delusions) that lasted 7 months. She was started on a small dose of olanzapine at the time of diagnosis, which resulted in the disappearance of all her psychotic symptoms. She has now been symptom free for the past 3 years. Which of the following treatment changes should be made first?

a. Her olanzapine should be decreased and then stopped if she remains symptom free.
b. Her olanzapine should be decreased, but not stopped.
c. Her olanzapine should be maintained at a constant level, but she can stretch out the time between her appointments with the psychiatrist.
d. Her diagnosis should be reexamined as she is likely not schizophrenic at all.
e. Her olanzapine should be switched to a long-acting depot antipsychotic medication such as haloperidol decanoate.

266. A 75-year-old man is being cared for in a hospice setting. He has widely spread prostatic carcinoma and is considered terminal. Which of the following psychiatric symptoms are seen in 90% of all terminal patients?

a. Delusions
b. Hallucinations
c. Flight of ideas
d. Anxiety
e. Depression

267. A 52-year-old man is seen by a psychiatrist in the emergency room because he is complaining about hearing and seeing miniature people who tell him to kill everyone in sight. He states that these symptoms developed suddenly during the past 48 hours, but that he has had them "on and off" for years. He states that he has never previously sought treatment for the symptoms, but that this episode is particularly bad. He denies the use of any illicit substances. The patient is alert and oriented to person, place, and time. His mental status examination is normal except for his auditory and visual hallucinations. His thought process is normal. His drug toxicology screen is positive for marijuana but no other substances. He is quite insistent that he needs to be "put away" in the hospital for the symptoms he is experiencing. Which of the following is the most likely diagnosis?

a. Substance-induced psychosis
b. Schizophrenia
c. Schizoaffective disorder
d. Schizophreniform disorder
e. Malingering

268. A 25-year-old man is brought to the physician after complaining about a visual hallucination of a transparent phantom of his own body. Which of the following specific syndromes is this patient most likely to be displaying?

a. Capgras syndrome
b. Lycanthropy
c. Cotard syndrome
d. Autoscopic psychosis
e. Folie à deux

Questions 269 to 275

Match the following vignettes with the diagnoses they best describe. Each lettered option may be used once, more than once, or not at all.

a. Brief psychotic disorder
b. Schizophreniform disorder
c. Schizophrenia
d. Schizoaffective disorder
e. Major depression with psychosis
f. Schizoid personality disorder
g. Schizotypal personality disorder

269. A 21-year-old man is brought to the psychiatrist by his parents. They state that for the previous year, he has been withdrawn, apathetic, and somewhat suspicious of his friends. For the past week, he has isolated himself in his room because he states that there are voices telling him that his friends are going to hurt him.

270. A 36-year-old woman presents to the physician with hallucinations of feeling that her skin is burning. Her speech is somewhat disorganized and difficult to follow. Her husband states that this behavior has been occurring for the past week, ever since she was told of a car crash that killed her daughter.

271. A 39-year-old man is referred to a psychiatrist by his employment assistance program, after he began having trouble on his job. The patient states that his stress level is very high ever since he was promoted to his new job as manager of his computer department. He states that before the promotion, he was quite happy off in his cubicle interacting with no one but the computer all day long. He had that job for over 15 years, and did it well.

272. A 24-year-old graduate student is shunned by his fellow graduate students because he is so "odd." He discusses topics like whether or not crystals are real forms of galactic communication, and wonders out loud about the wiring in the building where he works as to whether it has special meaning in its architecture. The student denies having any kind of hallucination.

273. A 26-year-old woman presents to the emergency room accompanied by her fiancée. He notes that she has been acting increasingly strangely over the past 3 weeks. She states that the TV is beaming messages directly into her brain, and that she can't understand why he can't hear the messages too. Her hygiene has also gotten poorer, and she has not taken a shower in the past week because the water might "turn into acid."

274. A 32-year-old man presents to the emergency room complaining of depressed mood and "odd" thinking. He notes that people from the CIA are watching his apartment and this is very depressing to him. This is the third episode of this kind of behavior in this man's history. Four weeks later, he has a return visit to the emergency room complaining of the CIA, but his mood symptoms have resolved.

275. A 48-year-old woman comes to the psychiatrist because she "must be the worst person in the world." She gives a 2-month history of becoming increasingly sad. She is having trouble sleeping and has lost 10 lb without trying. Two weeks prior to the visit, she started to become obsessed with the notion that she is a bad person and that a cancer was eating her alive from the inside out.

Schizophrenia and Other Psychotic Disorders

Answers

238. The answer is c. *(Kaplan and Sadock, pp 1046-1047.)* The patient has neuroleptic malignant syndrome (NMS), a life-threatening complication of antipsychotic treatment. The symptoms include muscular rigidity and dystonia, akinesia, mutism, obtundation, and agitation. The autonomic symptoms include high fever, sweating, and increased blood pressure and heart rate. Mortality rates are reported to be 10% to 20%. In addition to supportive medical treatment, the most commonly used medications for the condition are dantrolene (Dantrium) followed by bromocriptine (Parlodel), although amantadine is sometimes used. Bromocriptine and amantadine possess direct dopamine receptor agonist effects and may serve to overcome the antipsychotic-induced dopamine receptor blockade. Dantrolene is a direct muscle relaxant.

239 and 240. The answers are 239-c, 240-c. *(Kaplan and Sadock, p 490.)* Tardive dyskinesia (TD) is characterized by involuntary choreoathetoid movements of the face, trunk, and extremities. Tardive dyskinesia is associated with prolonged use of medications that block dopamine receptors, most commonly antipsychotic medications. Typical antipsychotic medications (such as perphenazine) and, in particular, high-potency drugs carry the highest risk of TD. Atypical antipsychotics are thought to be less likely to cause this disorder.

241. The answer is d. *(Kaplan and Sadock, p 476.)* Factors weighting toward a good prognosis in schizophrenia include: late onset of the disease, obvious precipitating factors/stressors, an acute onset, good premorbid functioning, the presence of mood disorder symptoms, the patient being married, a family history of mood disorders, good support systems, and the presence of positive symptoms (as opposed to negative symptoms).

242. The answer is a. *(Kaplan and Sadock, p 489.)* The use of a benzodiazepine and a high-potency antipsychotic has several advantages. While the antipsychotic treats the psychosis without a lot of anticholinergic side effects, the benzodiazepine reduces the amount of antipsychotic needed and protects the patient against dystonic reactions. Clozapine or fluphenazine decanoate would never be given in an acute setting.

243. The answer is e. *(Kaplan and Sadock, p 490.)* If a patient has not responded well to a conventional dopamine receptor antagonist (first-generation antipsychotic), it is unlikely the patient will respond well to another. It is better to switch to a low dose of serotonin dopamine antagonists (second-generation antipsychotic). It is too early in the treatment of this patient (ie, only one antipsychotic tried) to give up on them all together and go to clozapine, which has significant monitoring and the possibility of life-threatening reactions involved.

244. The answer is e. *(Kaplan and Sadock, pp 537-538.)* This patient is presenting with a major depression with psychotic features. For over 2 weeks (the minimum for the diagnosis), the patient has been complaining of anhedonia, crying, anergia, decreased concentration, 25-lb weight loss, and insomnia with early morning awakening. She also has somatic delusions that are mood congruent and an auditory hallucination. The presence of psychotic phenomena that follow a clear mood disorder picture makes the diagnosis of major depression with psychotic features the most likely.

245. The answer is c. *(Jacobson and Jacobson, pp 53-55.)* Schizophreniform disorder and chronic schizophrenia differ only in the duration of the symptoms and the fact that the impaired social or occupational functioning associated with chronic schizophrenia is not required to diagnose schizophreniform disorder. As with schizophrenia, schizophreniform disorder is characterized by the presence of delusions, hallucinations, disorganized thoughts and speech, and negative symptoms. The total duration of the illness, including prodromal and residual phases, is at least 1 month and less than 6 months. Approximately one-third of patients diagnosed with schizophreniform disorder experience a full recovery, while the rest progress to schizophrenia and schizoaffective disorder.

Depending on the predominance of particular symptoms, five subtypes of schizophrenia are recognized: paranoid, disorganized, catatonic, residual, and undifferentiated. The man in the question presents with the classic symptoms of paranoid schizophrenia. This subtype of schizophrenia is characterized by prominent hallucinations and delusional ideations with a relative preservation of affect and cognitive functions. Delusions are usually grandiose or persecutory or both, organized around a central coherent theme. Hallucinations, usually auditory, are frequent and related to the delusional theme. Anxiety, anger, argumentativeness, and aloofness are often present. Paranoid schizophrenia tends to develop later in life and is associated with a better prognosis.

246. The answer is a. *(Jacobson and Jacobson, pp 55-56.)* The main feature of delusional disorder is the presence of one or more nonbizarre delusions without deterioration of psychosocial functioning and in the absence of bizarre or odd behavior. Auditory and visual hallucinations, if present, are not prominent and are related to the delusional theme. Tactile and olfactory hallucinations may also be present if they are incorporated in the delusional system (such as feeling insects crawling over the skin in delusions of infestation). Subtypes of delusional disorder include erotomanic, grandiose, jealous, persecutory, and somatic (delusions of being infested with parasites, of emitting a bad odor, of having AIDS). Delusional disorder usually manifests in middle or late adult life and has a fluctuating course with periods of remissions and relapses. The patient in the vignette clearly demonstrates persecutory delusions, but no hallucinations or other bizarre or odd behavior, which makes her diagnosis delusional disorder.

247. The answer is a. *(Kaplan and Sadock, p 477.)* The essential characteristics of the disorganized type of schizophrenia are disorganized speech and behavior, flat or inappropriate affect, great functional impairment, and inability to perform basic activities such as showering or preparing meals. Grimacing, along with silly and odd behavior and mannerisms, is common. Hallucinations and delusions, if present, are fragmented and not organized according to a coherent theme. This subtype is associated with poor premorbid functions, early insidious onset, and a progressive course without remissions. The patient has obviously had the disorder too long for the diagnosis to be schizophreniform, and the absence of mood symptoms makes a diagnosis of bipolar disorder or schizoaffective disorder unlikely. Patients with a delusional disorder do not generally have such a marked impairment in affect or function.

248. The answer is d. (*Kaplan and Sadock, p 477.*) Catatonic schizophrenia is characterized by marked psychomotor disturbances including prolonged immobility, posturing, extreme negativism (the patient actively resists any attempts made to change his or her position) or waxy flexibility (the patient maintains the position in which he or she is placed), mutism, echolalia (repetition of words said by another person), and echopraxia (repetition of movements made by another person). Periods of immobility and mutism can alternate with periods of extreme agitation (catatonic excitement).

249. The answer is a. (*Kaplan and Sadock, pp 501-504.*) Schizoaffective disorder is diagnosed when the required criteria for schizophrenia are met (delusions, hallucination, disorganized speech or behavior, and/or negative symptoms; duration of the disturbance, including prodromal and residual period, of at least 6 months with at least 1 month of active symptoms) and the patient experiences at some point in the course of the illness a major depressive episode or a manic episode. The man in the question meets all these criteria. Delusional disorder is not accompanied by a decline in functionality or significant affective symptoms. Individuals with schizoid personality disorder do not experience psychotic symptoms. Bipolar disorder is differentiated from schizoaffective disorder by the absence of periods of psychosis accompanied by prominent affective symptoms.

250. The answer is b. (*Kaplan and Sadock, pp 501-504.*) Schizoaffective disorder is diagnosed when the required criteria for schizophrenia are met (delusions, hallucination, disorganized speech or behavior, and/or negative symptoms; duration of the disturbance, including prodromal and residual period, of at least 6 months with at least 1 month of active symptoms) and the patient experiences, at some point in the course of the illness, a major depressive episode or a manic episode. The woman in this question meets all these criteria. She has continuing psychotic symptomatology, interspersed with episodes of a major mood disorder. Notably, she has never had the mood symptoms without the psychotic symptoms, ruling out major depression with psychosis as the diagnosis. Delusional disorder is not accompanied by decline in function or significant affective symptoms. Individuals with schizoid personality disorder do not experience psychotic symptoms. Bipolar disorder is differentiated from schizoaffective disorder in that bipolar disorder would never have periods of psychosis in the *absence* of prominent affective symptoms, as this woman does.

251. The answer is a. (*Kaplan and Sadock, p 509.*) This patient is suffering from an erotomanic delusion—the delusion of having a special relationship with another person, often someone famous.

252 to 256. The answers are 252-d, 253-b, 254-c, 255-e, 256-f. (*Kaplan and Sadock, pp 507-508, 510, 1076.*) Persecutory and jealous delusions are probably the most frequently seen by psychiatrists. Patients with the persecutory subtype of delusion are convinced they are being harassed or harmed by others. Those with the jealous type are often verbally and physically abusive to those involved in the delusion (the wife in this case). These delusions are very difficult to treat. The erotomanic delusion consists of the patient believing that someone (usually someone of perceived higher status, like a TV star) is in love with them. Somatic type delusions cause the sufferer to believe that they are afflicted with some physical disorder, and this belief is fixed (unlike hypochondriasis, in which the sufferer can be relieved of the belief that something is wrong, if only temporarily). Grandiose delusions have the patient believing that there is something special about him/her, such as God giving special messages. Mixed delusions combine several types of delusions in one presentation. Unspecified delusions are those reserved for presentations that cannot be characterized by the previous types. One example is Capgras syndrome, which is a delusion in which the patient believes that familiar people have been replaced by imposters.

257. The answer is b. (*Kaplan and Sadock, p 1053.*) There is strong evidence that without continuous treatment, virtually all schizophrenic patients relapse within 12 to 24 months. Injectable depot medications such as haloperidol decanoate and fluphenazine decanoate are effective in decreasing the rate of relapse in patients who are not compliant with oral medication.

258. The answer is d. (*Kaplan and Sadock, pp 501-504; Moore and Jefferson, pp 125-126.*) Brief psychotic disorder is characterized by the sudden appearance of delusions, hallucinations, and disorganized speech or behavior, usually following a severe stressor. The episode lasts at least 1 day and less than 1 month and is followed by full spontaneous remission. For the woman in the question, the psychotic episode was clearly precipitated by the death of her children. Schizophreniform disorder is differentiated from brief psychotic disorder by temporal factors (in schizophreniform disorder, symptoms are required to last more than 1 month) and lack of association with a stressor. Posttraumatic stress disorder has a more chronic course and is characterized by affective, dissociative, and behavioral symptoms.

259. The answer is a. (*Kaplan and Sadock, p 468.*) Schizophrenia affects 1% of the adult population. The incidence is comparable in all societies. The 1-year incidence rate is 0.2 per 1000.

260. The answer is d. (*Kaplan and Sadock, p 476.*) Factors predicting a good outcome in schizophrenia include age at onset of 20 to 25, possibly female gender, middle to high socioeconomic status, and a stable occupational record. Other adverse social factors are missing, and the family history is one of affective disorder, not schizophrenia. In addition, precipitating factors are usually present, and the onset of the disease is rapid, not insidious, in patients with good-outcome schizophrenia.

261. The answer is d. (*Jacobson and Jacobson, pp 112, 280.*) Amphetamine intoxication can result in a psychosis very closely resembling acute paranoid schizophrenia, with symptoms including paranoid delusions and visual hallucinations. Some investigators believe that prominent visual hallucinations and a relative absence of thought disorder are more characteristic of amphetamine psychosis, but other investigators believe the symptoms are indistinguishable. Other drugs that produce psychoses similar to schizophrenia include phencyclidine (PCP) and lysergic acid diethylamide (LSD).

262. The answer is d. (*Kaplan and Sadock, p 910.*) Auditory hallucinations are quite common in psychiatrically caused psychoses, but the rest of the items on the options list speak to the opposite, that is, a medical cause for the psychosis. Other signs that point to a medical cause could be other mental status signs such as speech, movement or gait disorders, problems with alertness, memory, concentration, or orientation, and a concurrent substance abuse history or medical problem.

263. The answer is a. (*Kaplan and Sadock, pp 467-468, 475.*) Frieda Fromm-Reichmann followed the interpersonal school founded by Harry Stack Sullivan and believed that schizophrenia was the outcome of an inadequate mother–child relationship in which the mother was aloof, overly protective, or hostile. She postulated that faulty mothering leads to anxiety and distrust of others, causing people who develop schizophrenia to withdraw from interpersonal exchanges. This theory has been discredited by recent research that supports the notion that schizophrenia is a brain disorder caused by the convergence of multiple environmental and genetic factors. However, subsequent study of the affect of expressed emotion (family members expressive of hostility and overly controlling) do show that this behavior leads to an increase in relapse rates.

264. The answer is d. (*Moore and Jefferson, p 434.*) Self-induced water intoxication should always be considered in the differential diagnosis of confusional states and seizures in schizophrenic patients. As many as 20% of patients with a diagnosis of schizophrenia drink excessive amounts of water. At least 4% of these patients suffer from chronic hyponatremia and recurrent acute water intoxication. Medications that cause excessive water retention, such as lithium and carbamazepine, can aggravate the symptomatology.

265. The answer is a. (*Kaplan and Sadock, p 489.*) This patient has had one single episode of psychosis and has remained symptom free on her medication for over 3 years. Guidelines state that such a patient should be discontinued from antipsychotic medication, although a gradual reduction in the medication first, along with more frequent visits to the psychiatrist during this time, should be implemented to minimize the risk of relapse. In addition, it is recommended that the patient and family be encouraged to develop early intervention strategies prior to medication discontinuation, should a relapse occur.

266. The answer is a. (*Kaplan and Sadock, p 1366.*) Delusions are an extremely common symptom of terminally ill patients, occurring in 90% of them. The delusions may be reversed if their cause is treatable (eg, a delusion occurring secondary to a medication intoxication). The delusions are usually responsive to antipsychotic medications. Symptoms of anxiety and depression may also occur, but not with such overwhelming frequency as is seen with delusions.

267. The answer is e. (*Jacobson and Jacobson, pp 153, 156, 159.*) This patient is probably malingering. It is quite likely that if he is admitted, he will be found to have some secondary-gain reason for wanting to be in the hospital (eg, to avoid the legal system). It is unlikely at his age that he would suddenly become ill with schizophreniform disorder, schizophrenia, or schizoaffective disorder. The rather simplistic description of hallucinations in an otherwise clear sensorium and the absence of a disordered thought process also arise the suspicion of malingering. Although the patient does have marijuana in his system, its presence serves to highlight that this patient is being less than truthful rather than suggesting a substance-induced psychosis, since it is unlikely marijuana alone would cause such symptoms.

268. The answer is d. (*Ebert et al, p 304.*) Autoscopic psychosis has, as its main symptom, the visual hallucination of a transparent phantom of one's own body. Capgras syndrome (delusion of doubles) is a fixed belief that familiar persons have been replaced by identical imposters who behave exactly like the original person. Lycanthropy is the delusion that the person is a werewolf or other animal. Cotard syndrome is the false perception of having lost everything, including money, status, strength, health, and internal organs. Folie à deux is a shared psychotic disorder in which one person develops psychotic symptoms similar to the ones a long-term partner has been experiencing.

269 to 275. The answers are 269-c, 270-a, 271-f, 272-g, 273-b, 274-d, 275-e. (*Ebert et al, pp 261-303.*) The young man in the first vignette in this series is suffering from schizophrenia. He has had a prodromal period lasting a year (longer than the 6 months of symptoms necessary for this diagnosis) with 1 week of frankly psychotic behavior (auditory hallucinations). The woman in the next question is suffering from a brief psychotic disorder. This disorder may occur in a patient with no previous prodromal symptoms and no prior history of psychotic behavior, after a severe trauma, such as occurred with this patient. Note that the age of this patient also makes it unlikely that this is a first break of schizophrenia. The 39-year-old man in the third vignette is suffering from a schizoid personality disorder. Note that he shows no evidence of psychosis, and shows up to the psychiatrist because he cannot handle the interpersonal interactions required of his new job. He was quite happy in his cubicle, working alone, with no friends. This is the hallmark of a schizoid personality disorder. The student in question 272 has a schizotypal personality disorder. Note the odd behavior, which is enough to cause his fellow graduate students to avoid him. There is no mention of a real psychosis, and it appears that this behavior has been life-long, making a personality disorder diagnosis appropriate. The 26-year-old woman in question 273 has a schizophreniform disorder. Note the frankly psychotic symptoms—that of the delusion of a TV beaming messages into her brain, and the auditory hallucinations of the messages themselves. In addition, her hygiene has gotten markedly poorer. All of this occurs within a 3-week time frame with no mention of a sudden stressor. If this behavior continues for 6 months, she would have to be diagnosed as a schizophrenic. The man in question 274 has a schizoaffective disorder. Note that he has a combination of depressed mood and "odd" thinking. He has clear paranoid delusions. During a return visit to the emergency room, he also has evidence of psychotic symptoms but no mood symptoms, making this a diagnosis of schizoaffective disorder. The woman in the last vignette in this series has a major depression with psychosis. Note the history of depressed symptoms occurring first, in the absence of psychotic symptoms, with psychotic symptoms developing secondarily as the depression worsens. Note also that this patient's delusions are congruent with her mood—that is, they are of some very depressing content instead of being just frankly bizarre.

Psychotherapies

Questions

276. A 28-year-old woman comes to the psychiatrist for help with her fear of flying. She states that for as long as she can remember, she has been afraid to fly. She has been able to do so, despite her fear, but she reports feeling trapped and extremely anxious each time she must do so. In addition, she has a great deal of anticipatory anxiety about any upcoming flight. She has recently taken a new job that requires flying for business at least twice per month and so would like to rid herself of this fear. Which of the following treatment options is optimal for this young woman?

a. Identifying the patient's maladaptive assumptions about flying
b. Individual psychodynamic psychotherapy
c. Group therapy with patients also afraid of flying
d. Systematic desensitization
e. Alprazolam prn before flying

277. A 45-year-old man is diagnosed as having diabetes and will require insulin. His physician explains the use of the medication and tells the patient that he will need to be seen at frequent intervals until his glucose levels come under good control. The patient has always been somewhat hostile with the physician, but upon hearing this news, he says angrily, "You doctors are always the same! You always want control—of my time, of my money, and now of my every action!" As far as the physician knows, this patient has never had an unpleasant encounter with a physician before. Which of the following is the most likely explanation for the patient's reaction to his doctor?

a. The patient is becoming delusional.
b. The patient is experiencing transference to this authority figure.
c. The patient is splitting.
d. The patient is becoming manic.
e. The patient is anticipating being rejected by his physician.

Questions 278 and 279

278. A 45-year-old woman comes to the psychiatrist requesting help in coping with her life. The patient states both of her parents have recently been diagnosed with cancer and her husband has just instituted divorce proceedings. She states she feels overwhelmed and anxious, with bouts of crying and panic attacks. Which one of the following therapies should be offered to this patient?

a. Medication management
b. Psychoanalytic psychotherapy
c. Psychodynamic psychotherapy
d. Family therapy
e. Supportive psychotherapy

279. In the above patient, which of the following signs or symptoms should push the physician to recommend insight-oriented psychodynamic psychotherapy once the patient's life had returned to a less-stressful state?

a. Poor reality testing
b. High tolerance for frustration
c. Organically based cognitive dysfunction
d. Low intelligence
e. Poor impulse control

280. A 32-year-old woman presented to the psychiatric emergency room after a suicide attempt in which she swallowed a bottle of aspirin. On the inpatient unit it was noted that she was stealing needles and injecting feces under her skin to cause infections. She has a long history of multiple surgical procedures for unclear reasons. Which of the following guidelines is most useful for treatment of patients with this disorder?

a. Appoint a psychiatrist as the primary gatekeeper for all medical and psychiatric treatments.
b. Regular interdisciplinary team meetings to control splitting.
c. Aggressively and directly confront this patient's behavior and her illness.
d. Discharge the patient from the hospital as soon as possible.
e. Use invasive diagnostic procedures early to get a quick diagnosis of any presenting physical signs or symptoms.

281. What is the most common reason that psychotherapy for personality disorders is so difficult to carry out successfully?

a. The traits are often ego-dystonic.
b. The patients are usually too sick to use psychotherapy.
c. These disorders respond better to medication than to psychotherapy.
d. The patients often see the source of their problems in others, not themselves.
e. The patients do not have the ego strength for weekly meetings.

282. A patient in psychodynamic therapy has been coming late to the last few sessions and complaining in the sessions that he has nothing to talk about. His therapist points out that up until several weeks ago they were making very rapid progress into uncovering some of the difficult thoughts and feelings the patient had about his parents. What therapeutic principle best exemplifies the recent changes in the patient's behavior?

a. Countertransference
b. Ego strength
c. Abreaction
d. Projective identification
e. Resistance

283. A 24-year-old woman with bulimia joins an eating disorder support group on the advice of her psychiatrist. After years of being deeply ashamed of her disorder and keeping it secret, she is relieved to hear that others in the group have binged and purged as she has. Which of the following terms best describes this phenomenon, which is common in self-help groups?

a. Universalization
b. Group cohesion
c. Multiple transference
d. Shared belief system
e. Validation

284. A 22-year-old student is in therapy because he has a long history of chaotic interpersonal relationships, episodes of psychosis, and multiple hospitalizations. He has attempted suicide three times, mostly precipitated by his feeling overwhelmed in some social setting. One session, he comes to his therapist greatly upset and anxious because he forgot to study some material that will be on an upcoming examination. The therapist reminds the patient that he has done well on previous examinations and suggests that she help him devise a study plan for the time the patient has left before the test. Such an intervention is commonly used in which of the following therapies?

a. Psychoanalysis
b. Object relation psychotherapy
c. Cognitive-behavioral therapy
d. Supportive psychotherapy
e. Interpersonal psychotherapy

Questions 285 and 286

285. A 37-year-old man comes to the psychiatrist for treatment of a depressed mood. The patient has anhedonia, anergia, decreased concentration, obsessive ruminations of guilt, insomnia, and a 5-lb weight loss over the past 2 weeks. He avoids going out in public secondary to the belief that people won't like him. In the psychiatrist's office, he was helped to verbalize the fact that whenever he met new people, his immediate reaction was to believe that these people could see he was "a loser." This last is a verbalization of which kind of behavior, often seen in patients with this diagnosis?

a. Automatic thought
b. Delusion
c. Obsession
d. Avoidance
e. Modeling

286. In the vignette above, the patient's verbalization that "when people see me they think I'm a loser" is most often used directly in the context of which kind of therapy?

a. Psychodynamic psychotherapy
b. Family therapy
c. Cognitive therapy
d. Behavioral therapy
e. Supportive psychotherapy

287. A 45-year-old woman comes to a therapist with the chief complaint of feeling depressed. The therapist asks the patient to talk about her experiences, both in daily life and in the past. As the therapy progresses, the patient realizes that much of her depressive emotion comes from her feelings of abandonment as a child, when her mother was hospitalized for a long illness and was thus unavailable. The patient sees the therapist once a week. The therapist uses primarily clarification, confrontation, and interpretation as tools. Which of the following therapies is this patient most likely undergoing?

a. Dynamic psychotherapy
b. Cognitive therapy
c. Behavioral therapy
d. Psychoanalysis
e. Experiential-humanistic psychotherapy

Questions 288 to 294

Match the correct defense mechanism with each patient's actions. Each lettered option may be used once, more than once, or not at all.

a. Distortion
b. Repression
c. Reaction formation
d. Sublimation
e. Somatization
f. Intellectualization
g. Suppression
h. Isolation of affect
i. Introjection
j. Projection
k. Identification with the aggressor
l. Projective identification
m. Denial
n. Displacement

288. A patient starts complaining of chest pain and coughing whenever her therapist confronts her. She insists, however, that she is not at all distressed or angry.

289. A woman feels jealous and hurt when, at a family gathering, her husband flirts with her younger cousin. She makes a conscious decision to put her feelings aside and to wait for a more appropriate moment to confront her husband and convey her emotions.

290. A young man gets into an argument with his teacher. Although he is very upset, he remains silent as she chastises him severely and calls him a failure as a student. Once he gets home from school, the young man picks a fight with his younger brother over nothing and begins screaming at him.

291. A 34-year-old man is deeply envious of his younger but much more successful brother. Although it is difficult for him to admit, he believes the younger brother was their parents' favorite as well. He tells his friends that his younger brother is envious of his good looks and successes with women, even though there is some evidence that this is not so.

292. A 28-year-old woman is in psychotherapy for a long-standing depressed mood and poor self-esteem. One day during the session, the therapist yawns because she is very tired, though she is interested in what the patient has to say. The patient immediately bursts into tears, saying that the therapist must be bored and uninterested in her and must have been so for quite some time.

293. A man who, as a child, was beaten by his parents for every small infraction nonetheless idealizes them and describes them as "good parents who did not spoil their children." He is baffled and angry when he is ordered to start parenting classes after the school nurse reports that his children consistently come to school with bruises.

294. A 52-year-old man is hospitalized after a severe myocardial infarction. On the second day in the hospital, when his physician comes by on rounds, the patient insists on jumping out of bed and doing several push-ups to show the physician that "they can't keep a good man down—there is nothing wrong with me!"

Questions 295 to 297

Match each of the following vignettes with the type of psychotherapy that is being employed. Each lettered option may be used once, more than once, or not at all.

a. Insight-oriented psychodynamic psychotherapy
b. Supportive psychotherapy
c. Short-term psychodynamic psychotherapy
d. Psychoanalysis
e. Cognitive therapy
f. Behavioral therapy
g. Experiential-humanistic therapy
h. Eclectic or integrated (mixed) therapy

295. A 24-year-old man comes to the therapist after being discharged from the hospital following treatment for a psychotic episode. The patient is currently stable on antipsychotic medication. He visits the therapist every other week and during the sessions he describes troubles in his relationship with his parents and in finding a job, and his occasional hallucinations. The therapist responds empathically to his difficulties and occasionally makes a suggestion as to how he might handle his job search more effectively.

296. A 22-year-old man comes to the therapist with the chief complaint of incredible anxiety during multiple-choice examinations. He reports that he becomes unable to focus, begins to sweat, and is unable to retrieve the information he knows he has learned. During sessions, the therapist hooks the patient up to a machine that measures galvanic skin response and trains the patient in relaxation techniques.

297. A 35-year-old woman comes to the therapist because she feels pessimistic about her life and is unable to enjoy her successful job and two healthy children. She has multiple symptoms, including feeling chronically depressed, anxious, phobic, and compulsive. She has a history of childhood sexual abuse. She notes that these problems have been long standing. The therapist teaches the patient relaxation skills and begins to have her talk about her childhood sexual abuse.

298. A 48-year-old woman comes to the psychiatrist because she has an overwhelming fear of spiders. She has had this fear her entire life, but it has increased now secondary to living in a wooded area where there are greater numbers of them. She wishes to get rid of this phobia. Which of the following actions should the psychiatrist take next?

a. Prescribe alprazolam
b. Prescribe bupropion
c. Prescribe propranolol
d. Have the patient create a hierarchical list of feared situations involving spiders
e. Engage the patient in psychodynamic psychotherapy to get at the root of her arachnophobia

299. A patient in psychotherapy is always anxious to please. Recently, he stated that he has begun to feel frightened in the presence of the therapist and that he has had fantasies about the analyst attacking him. Subsequently, the patient talks about his father and his lifelong struggle to please him at any cost. After listening to these comments, the therapist says that the patient's fantasies about him appear to be closely connected with the patient's way of relating to his father. The therapist also says that the passive and compliant relationship the patient has with his idealized father may represent a reaction to his fear of his father's retaliation. These comments best represent which kind of therapeutic intervention?

a. Confrontation
b. Interpretation
c. Clarification
d. Desensitization
e. Flooding

300. A 29-year-old woman is in psychodynamic psychotherapy for a long-standing inability to have close and meaningful relationships. During her sessions with the therapist, she often comes 10 minutes late or misses sessions altogether. At the beginning of the next session after a session has been missed, the therapist points out this behavior to the patient. These comments best represent which kind of therapeutic intervention?

a. Confrontation
b. Interpretation
c. Clarification
d. Desensitization
e. Flooding

301. The parents of a 20-year-old schizophrenic are having difficulty dealing with their son's decline in function. Once a good student with friends and a social life, the son now spends his days barricaded in his room, mumbling to himself, or watching the street with binoculars. Which of the following family interventions would be most helpful in this situation?

a. Teaching the parents about reducing expressed emotions in the family's interactions
b. Unmasking the family game and freeing the identified patient from the role of symptom bearer
c. Encouraging the parents to openly discuss their feelings of loss and disappointment with their son
d. Discussing the secondary gains provided by the son's symptoms
e. Discussing the parents' marital problems and how the son's disorder affects them

302. A 27-year-old man comes to the physician with the chief complaint of premature ejaculation. He has been married for 4 months but has been unable to consummate the marriage because of his sexual problem. No organic cause for his premature ejaculation was found on work-up. Which of the following treatments will be most helpful for the man's premature ejaculation?

a. Exploration of the husband's relationship with his domineering mother
b. Discussion of the wife's unexpressed masochistic fantasies
c. Interpretation of the husband's dreams
d. Squeeze technique and stop-and-start technique
e. Instructing the husband to masturbate several times a day with the goal to reach an orgasm as fast as possible

303. A 49-year-old man comes to the doctor with high blood pressure and anxiety. Preferring to try something other than medication at first, the patient agrees to try another approach. He is attached to an apparatus that measures skin temperature and emits a tone proportional to the temperature. Which of the following techniques is being used with this patient?

a. Hypnosis
b. Progressive muscle relaxation
c. Autogenic techniques
d. Placebo
e. Biofeedback

304. A high school teacher is respected and loved by both his students and his colleagues because he can easily defuse tense moments with an appropriate light remark and he always seems to be able to find something funny in any situation. Which of the following defense mechanisms is this man using?

a. Displacement
b. Denial
c. Reaction formation
d. Humor
e. Suppression

Questions 305 to 307

For each patient, select the one most appropriate therapeutic option. Each lettered option may be used once, more than once, or not at all.

a. Psychoanalysis
b. Brief individual psychotherapy
c. Cognitive therapy
d. Behavioral therapy
e. Family therapy
f. Group therapy

305. A young woman with no previous psychiatric history develops an incapacitating fear of driving after being involved in a minor automobile accident.

306. A 16-year-old girl begins acting out sexually and skipping school. These symptoms coincide with the onset of frequent arguments between her parents, who have been threatening marital separation.

307. An intelligent 25-year-old single woman who has a successful career complains of multiple failed relationships with men, unhappiness, and a wish to sort out her life. A previous experience in individual psychotherapy was somewhat helpful.

308. A 29-year-old woman comes to a cognitive therapist with a 6-month history of sudden feelings that she is going to die. The patient reports that during these episodes her pulse races, she feels short of breath, and she gets chest pain. She notes that she feels like she is going to die on the spot and therefore has begun to restrict her movement outside the house so that she can remain near a phone in case she needs to call an ambulance. Which of the following treatment interventions should the therapist employ first to begin to help this patient with her problem?

a. Taking the patient to a crowded place and preventing her escape until her anxiety has peaked
b. Teaching the patient to hyperventilate as soon as she starts feeling anxious
c. Educating the patient about the harmless nature of the physical symptoms experienced during a panic attack
d. Taking the patient through a series of imaginary exposures in the therapist's office
e. Replying empathically to the patient about the suffering that must be endured with panic attacks

309. A physician with a very busy practice feels satisfied and fulfilled when he can make a difference in the lives of his patients. Which of the following defense mechanisms is being used, according to psychoanalytic theory?

a. Reaction formation
b. Altruism
c. Sublimation
d. Asceticism
e. Idealization

310. An 18-year-old girl comes to the psychiatrist because she pulls out her hair in patches when she is anxious or upset. She is taught to make a tight fist whenever she has this impulse rather than pull out her hair. Which of the following techniques is this?

a. Habit reversal training
b. Extinction
c. Simple conditioning
d. Flooding
e. Desensitization

311. A 34-year-old man comes to the psychiatrist complaining of marital problems, which seemed to have begun just after the death of his mother. In therapy, it is discovered that the patient had an intensively ambivalent relationship with his mother. However, when he discusses his mother, the patient appears unemotional and detached. Which of the following defense mechanisms is this patient using?

a. Projection
b. Isolation of affect
c. Splitting
d. Reaction formation
e. Projective identification

312. A 32-year-old man comes to a therapist with the chief complaint of not being able to have a successful and happy relationship with a woman. During the course of the therapy, it becomes obvious that the patient has deep-seated anger against women, even though he is consciously unaware of it. Around the time that this interpretation is being worked on in therapy, the patient begins to go to bars and drink to excess—something he had not previously done. When confronted about the behavior, he denies that this has anything to do with what is going on in the therapy, though the therapist does not believe this to be true. Which of the following best describes this patient's new behavior?

a. The patient is acting out.
b. The patient is acting in.
c. The patient is experiencing a new onset of substance abuse disorder.
d. The patient is seeking to find a relationship.
e. The patient is in a fugue state.

313. A young woman with obsessive-compulsive disorder has suffered from contamination fears for years, and now her hands are raw from so much washing. Her therapist takes her to the bathroom and asks her to touch the toilet seat. Afterward, he stops her from washing her hands. The patient's anxiety rapidly increases, and after a peak, declines. Which of the following is the name of this technique?

a. Exposure and response prevention
b. Desensitization
c. Counterconditioning
d. Operational conditioning
e. Functional behavioral analysis

Psychotherapies

Answers

276. The answer is d. (*Kaplan and Sadock, pp 953-954*.) Systematic desensitization is the treatment of choice for cases of clearly identifiable anxiety-provoking stimuli, like this woman's fear of flying. While alprazolam might well manage this patient's anxiety while in the air, it will not rid her of the phobia, nor will it help with her anticipatory anxiety about the flight. Systemic desensitization is a form of behavioral therapy, and involves three steps: relaxation training; hierarchical construction of anxiety provoking situations (for example, this patient's list might start with a low-anxiety situation, such as just thinking about a flight that is scheduled for 6 months away, and end with a high-anxiety situation, such as actually imagining herself sitting in an airplane while it experiences turbulence); and then desensitization to the stimulus (proceeding through the list from least anxiety-provoking through most anxiety-provoking while maintaining oneself in a deeply relaxed state).

277. The answer is b. (*Jacobson and Jacobson, p 500*.) Transference, according to the classical Freudian psychoanalytic theory, refers to the projection of feelings, thoughts, and attitudes once connected to important figures in the patient's past onto another important figure (often an authority figure). Transference causes patients to unconsciously reenact old scripts with new others (in this case, the physician). In this example, it is likely that this patient has experienced authority figures in his past who have attempted to control him in unwelcome and oppressive ways. Transference is not limited to a patient–psychiatrist relationship but can take place in any meaningful relationship. Verbal and nonverbal communication, overt behavioral patterns, omissions, and dreams are some of the ways transference manifests itself.

278. The answer is e. (*Kaplan and Sadock, pp 929-930*.) Supportive psychotherapy is generally the preferred choice in cases where patients are undergoing acute life crises and are feeling overwhelmed. This patient's current inability to cope with her daily life does not make it likely that any of the other forms of therapy listed in the options would be useful to her, and in fact, might cause her to regress still further. The goals of supportive therapy are to reduce patients' symptoms and help them better cope with their surrounding environments.

279. The answer is b. *(Kaplan and Sadock, p 930.)* Once the patient is no longer in an acutely stressful environment, a more insightful form of psychotherapy may be indicated if the patient still wishes to look at her life and her troubles with significant others. Insight-oriented psychotherapy requires a strongly motivated patient who can tolerate a great deal of frustration and has a good capacity for insight. These patients must be able to have good impulse control so that they may talk about their feelings without acting them out. Patients with low intelligence or with cognitive dysfunctions do not generally get benefit from this kind of therapy.

280. The answer is b. *(Kaplan and Sadock, p 664.)* The management of a patient with factitious disorder is difficult at best. Guidelines do exist, however. Harm to the patient must be minimized, which means all invasive tests and procedures should be kept to an absolute minimum. Splitting is common, so regular interdisciplinary team meetings are called for to manage these patients. Empathic, nonconfrontational, and face-saving maneuvers are generally preferred to aggressive or confrontational ones—the latter will most likely cause the patient to flee therapy. A primary care physician should be appointed gatekeeper of all treatment, medical and psychiatric.

281. The answer is d. *(Kaplan and Sadock, p 792.)* Although personality disorders cause considerable suffering for patients and people with whom they relate, these patients usually are oblivious to the fact that their characterological traits and maladaptive behaviors create and perpetuate their suffering (eg, their traits are ego-syntonic). On the contrary, these patients tend to blame others for their difficulties and deny that they have any problems. Relatives, friends, and coworkers usually have a much better understanding of the patient's dysfunctional traits than the patient has.

282. The answer is e. *(Kaplan and Sadock, p 192.)* Freud noticed that patients, in spite of their suffering and their overt desire to change, tended to cling to their symptoms and resisted the analyst's efforts to produce insight. He called these powerful internal forces that oppose change *resistance*. Resistance takes place at any point in the treatment, and particularly when unacceptable impulses or thoughts threaten to come into consciousness or a maladaptive defense mechanism is challenged. Resistance can manifest itself in many different ways, including withholding important thoughts from the analyst, falling silent during sessions, forgetting appointments, forgetting to pay the analyst, falling asleep during the session, and considering dropping out of treatment. The possible manifestations of resistance are countless and depend on the patient's defense mechanisms and personality. In other words, the patient's intrapsychic defenses manifest as resistance in the context of his or her interpersonal relationship with the analyst. Freud thought that resistance should be uncovered by the analyst but not challenged or interpreted. Modern analysts believe that resistance should be analyzed through the patient's free associations, supported by the analyst's observations.

283. The answer is a. (*Kaplan and Sadock, pp 934-940.*) Universalization, the awareness that the patient is not alone or unique in his or her suffering and that others share similar symptoms and difficulties, is a powerful healing factor in group therapy. The other items listed are also factors that facilitate the therapeutic group process. Group cohesion refers to the sense that the group is working together toward a common goal. Validation refers to the confirmation of the patient's reality through comparison with other group members' experiences and conceptualizations. Shared belief system refers to the notion that the group may come to have a framework of beliefs and ideas about issues that is common to everyone in the group. Multiple transference refers to the projections of feelings, thoughts, and wishes that belong to the patients' past experiences onto other group members and the group leaders.

284. The answer is d. (*Kaplan and Sadock, pp 929-930.*) Supportive psychotherapy is characterized by an emphasis on the nurturing, caring role of the therapist and a focus on current reality. Although insight-oriented strategies such as interpretations can be used, they are not the main therapeutic instruments. Supportive psychotherapy aims to foster and maintain a positive transference all the time in order to provide the patient with a consistently safe and secure atmosphere. Consolation, advice, reality testing, environmental manipulation, reassurance, and encouragement are strategies commonly used in supportive psychotherapy.

285. The answer is a. (*Kaplan and Sadock, p 959.*) Automatic thoughts (cognitive distortions) are thoughts that come between the time an event occurs externally and the person having the thought has an emotional reaction to the external event. For example, the belief that "I am so ugly" is an automatic thought that may occur in between a person complimenting another on their new dress (the external event) and the person in the dress exclaiming, "You must be crazy!" (Prompted by the emotional reaction of dismay.) Every psychopathological disorder has its own particular profile of distorted thoughts, which if known, can provide the framework for cognitive work to stop them.

286. The answer is c. (*Kaplan and Sadock, p 959.*) Once cognitive distortions are recognized and characterized, cognitive therapy is used to unravel them by testing them, identifying their maladaptive underlying assumptions, and testing the validity of those assumptions as well.

287. The answer is a. (*Ebert et al, pp 153-155.*) This patient is undergoing dynamic psychotherapy. Psychoanalysis would also use the understanding of the patient and the recreation of the past through clarification, confrontation, and interpretation, but typically the patient comes to the office more frequently than once per week, and often, though not always, the patient lies on a couch facing away from the therapist. A cognitive therapy would most likely focus on the negative worldview of this patient and attempt to restructure those thoughts. A behavioral therapist would most likely instruct the patient to change his/her behavior as an antecedent to recovery (such as exercising or another activity). An experiential-humanistic therapist would focus on developing a supportive and gratifying relationship with the patient to help provide the empathic responsiveness that was hypothesized as absent in the patient's past.

288 to 294. The answers are 288-e, 289-g, 290-n, 291-j, 292-a, 293-k, 294-m. (*Kaplan and Sadock, pp 202-203.*) In distortion, external reality is grossly rearranged to conform to internal needs. (For example, a patient states that her husband smiles broadly whenever she tells him of her obsessions, when in reality he is grimacing.)

Repression is the expelling or withholding of an idea or feeling from consciousness. (For example, a woman who has just been told she has a diagnosis of cancer goes home that evening and tells her husband that everything is fine. When confronted by this error, she seems genuinely surprised to hear the cancer diagnosis.) This defense differs from suppression by affecting conscious inhibition of impulses to the point of losing and not just postponing goals.

Reaction formation refers to the substitution of an unacceptable feeling or thought with its opposite. (For example, a person who is very angry at his wife brings home flowers for her.)

Sublimation is the achieving of impulse gratification and the retention of goals by altering a socially objectionable aim or object to a socially acceptable one. (For example, a person who wishes to be admired by everyone channels this behavior into doing charity work.) Sublimation allows instincts to be channeled rather than blocked or diverted. Sublimation is a mature defense, together with humor, altruism, asceticism, anticipation, and suppression.

Somatization is the conversion of psychic derivatives into bodily symptoms and reaction with somatic manifestations rather than psychic ones. (For example, a person who is extremely anxious about her relationship with her husband begins having abdominal pain when in his presence.)

Intellectualization is the excessive use of intellectual processes to avoid affective expression or experience. (A person who has gotten into a disagreement with his best friend spends hours objectively analyzing the conversation to understand what happened.)

Isolation of affect is the splitting or separation of an idea from the affect that accompanies it but that is repressed. (A person told that he has been fired from his long time place of employment appears unemotional about the fact.)

Introjection is the internalization of the qualities of an object. When used as a defense, it can obliterate the distinction between the subject and the object.

Projection is the perception of and reaction to unacceptable inner impulses and their derivatives as though they were outside the self. (A person who is angry at her friend is convinced that the friend is angry at her instead.)

Identification with the aggressor is the adoption of characteristics or behavior of the victim's aggressor as one's own. For example, it is not uncommon for the victim of child abuse to grow up to be an abusive parent him- or herself.

Projective identification occurs mostly in borderline personality disorder and consists of three steps: (1) an aspect of the self is projected onto someone else, (2) the projector tries to coerce the other person to identify with what has been projected, and (3) the recipient of the projection and the projector feel a sense of oneness or union. (A patient who is angry at her therapist becomes convinced that her therapist is angry at her. The patient then unconsciously acts in such a way that the therapist actually does begin to feel angry.)

Denial is the avoidance of awareness of some painful aspect of reality by negating sensory data.

Displacement refers to the shifting of an emotion or a drive from one object to another (eg, the shifting of unacceptable aggressive feelings toward one's parents to the family cat).

295 to 297. The answers are 295-b, 296-f, 297-h. (*Kaplan and Sadock, pp 953-968.*) The first patient is undergoing supportive psychotherapy, which is recognized by the *absence* of interpretations and the focus on helping the patient function in the real world. Concrete suggestions about improving functioning in the outside world (in this case, suggestions about a job search) are appropriate in this kind of therapy, which is often reserved for those patients with severe psychopathology. This kind of therapy is not considered curative but, rather, helps the patient maintain functioning at the current level without the worsening of the preexisting symptoms. Behavioral therapy, as practiced in question 296, is recognizable by the use of specific maneuvers (in this case, biofeedback) that will change the patient's behavior. In this instance, the patient was taught to control his own behavioral responses to anxiety, and thus presumably, he will do better on his multiple-choice exams. The patient in question 297 presents with a myriad of symptoms, all of which seem neurotic in nature (there is no psychosis or vegetative signs/symptoms of a major mood disorder). The history of sexual abuse and the long-standing history of these symptoms mean that the use of short-term therapy is unlikely to be helpful. Her many symptoms in many spheres indicate that an eclectic approach will offer the highest chance of improvement in the least amount of time.

298. The answer is d. (*Kaplan and Sadock, p 953.*) All behavioral treatments for phobias have in common exposure to the feared stimulus. Desensitization is based on the concept that when the feared stimulus is presented paired with a behavior that induces a state incompatible with anxiety (eg, deep muscle relaxation), the phobic stimulus loses its power to create anxiety (counterconditioning). This pairing of feared stimulus with a state incompatible with anxiety is called reciprocal inhibition. For desensitization to work, the anxiety elicited by the exposure has to be low. Treatment starts with exposure to stimuli that produce minimal anxiety and proceeds to stimuli with higher anxiety potential. Operant conditioning refers to the concept that behavior can be modified by changing the antecedents or the consequences of the behavior (contingency management). Flooding is another exposure-based treatment for phobia, based on extinction rather than counterconditioning. Reframing is an intervention used in family therapy and refers to giving a more acceptable meaning to a problematic behavior or situation.

299. The answer is b. *(Kaplan and Sadock, pp 926-928.)* Interpretations, the cornerstone of psychoanalytic psychotherapy, are explanatory statements made by the analyst that link a symptom, a behavior, or a feeling to its unconscious meaning. Ideally, interpretations help the patient become more aware of unconscious material that has come close to the surface. Confrontation and clarification are also used in psychoanalytic psychotherapy. In confrontation, the analyst points out to the patient something that the patient is trying to avoid. Clarification refers to putting together the information the patient has provided so far and reflecting it back to him or her in a more organized and succinct form. Flooding and desensitization are exposure techniques used in behavioral therapy.

300. The answer is a. *(Kaplan and Sadock, pp 926-928.)* As noted in question 268, confrontation as a therapeutic technique points out a particular behavior of the patient and tries to assign some meaning to it—typically that the patient is behaving in this manner in an attempt to avoid something. In this question, the patient is arriving late and missing appointments; the therapist, via confrontation, points out the behavior, then may note that such behavior is designed to remove the patient from therapy, perhaps because she is anxious, angry, or ambivalent about the therapy itself.

301. The answer is a. *(Kaplan and Sadock, pp 940-942.)* Family interventions that have been shown to be effective in the treatment of schizophrenic patients include teaching the family members about schizophrenia, emphasizing the importance of keeping interpersonal communication at a low emotional quotient (schizophrenic patients tend to relapse when exposed to the intense negative emotions of family members), and helping the family learn more adaptive ways to cope with stress. Discussing marital problems in front of the patient and sharing with the patient the distressing details of the parents' own struggles with his or her mental illness are bound to have negative effects. Uncovering the family game was one of the goals of systemic family therapy created by Selvini-Palazzoli and the Milan group. This model was accepted in the 1960s, when schizophrenia was considered the consequence of pathological parenting. In view of what is now known about schizophrenia's biological etiology, this theory is no longer considered valid.

302. The answer is d. *(Kaplan and Sadock, pp 701-705.)* Treatment of sexual dysfunctions relies on specific exercises, called sensate focus exercises, aimed at decreasing anxiety, to teach the couple to give and take pleasure without the pressure of performance, and to increase communication between partners. Furthermore, specific problems are addressed with special techniques. The squeeze technique, used to treat premature ejaculation, aims to raise the threshold of penile excitability by firmly squeezing the coronal ridge of the penis, so as to abruptly decrease the level of excitation, at the earliest sensation of impending orgasm. In the start-and-stop technique, stimulation is repeatedly stopped for a few seconds as soon as orgasm is impending and resumed when the level of excitability decreases.

303. The answer is e. *(Kaplan and Sadock, pp 949-953.)* Biofeedback refers to a therapeutic process in which information about the individual's physiological functions, such as blood pressure and heart rate, are monitored electronically and fed back to the individual by means of lights, sounds, or electronic gauges. Biofeedback allows individuals to control a variety of body responses and in turn to modulate pain and the physiological component of unpleasant emotions such as anxiety.

304. The answer is d. *(Kaplan and Sadock, pp 202-203.)* Individuals who use humor as a defense mechanism are able to make use of comedy to express feelings and thoughts with potentially disturbing content without experiencing subjective discomfort and without producing an unpleasant effect on others. Humor is a mature defense. Suppression is consciously or semi-consciously postponing attention to a conscious impulse or conflict. In suppression, discomfort is acknowledged but minimized.

305 to 307. The answers are 305-d, 306-e, 307-a. *(Kaplan and Sadock, pp 924-946.)* Behavioral therapy focuses on decreasing or ameliorating people's maladaptive behavior without theorizing about their inner conflicts. Behaviorists look for observable factors that have been learned or conditioned and can therefore be unlearned. In this example, the young woman has developed a phobia about driving, after being in an automobile accident. The behavioral therapy indicated here would be teaching the young woman relaxation exercises, then progressively desensitizing her to driving (the stimulus). Brief individual insight-oriented psychotherapy is characterized by a limited, predetermined number of sessions and the fact that the focus of the treatment remains on specific problematic areas in the life of the patient. Deep restructuring of the patient's psychological apparatus is not the goal of brief therapy. Highly motivated patients who function relatively well are good candidates for this type of therapy. Family therapy aims to improve the level of functioning of the family and the individual by altering the interactions among the family members. There are many different approaches to family therapy (psycho-dynamic, solution-oriented, narrative, systemic, strategic, structural, and transgenerational, to name only a few). Each school focuses on a particular aspect of the family dynamics and uses different techniques to obtain the desired results. For example, the structural school focuses on patterns of engagement-enmeshment and on family boundaries and hierarchies. The solution-oriented approach focuses on solutions and minimizes the importance of problems. Psychoanalytic psychotherapy is suited to patients with relatively good ego strengths, normal or superior intelligence, ability to abstract and think symbolically, and a genuine wish to understand themselves. Although Freud originally restricted the indications for psychoanalysis to patients with neuroses of a hysterical, phobic, or obsessive-compulsive nature, it is now felt that this type of therapy benefits a much larger range of patients, including patients with depressive and anxiety disorders, high-functioning borderline and narcissistic personality disorders, avoidant personality disorder, and obsessive-compulsive personality disorder. Psychoanalysis is also helpful for individuals who do not have a psychiatric diagnosis but experience problems with intimacy, interpersonal relationships, assertiveness, self-esteem, and so forth.

308. The answer is c. (*Kaplan and Sadock, p 596.*) The cognitive treatment of panic disorder focuses on the patient's tendency to make catastrophic interpretations about body sensations or states of mind. This approach includes a careful exploration of the patient's bodily symptoms before and during the panic attack and of the automatic thoughts that accompany them, in addition to an educational component focusing on the fact that, although terrifying, panic attack symptoms are not fatal. Other, more realistic interpretations of symptoms are discussed, and the patient is encouraged to come up with less catastrophic scenarios. ("Even if I have a panic attack in a store, the world does not end.") Exposure techniques are part of behavioral therapy. Empathy with the patient's suffering is a necessary element of all doctor–patient interactions, but in this case it does not represent a specific therapeutic technique.

309. The answer is b. (*Kaplan and Sadock, pp 202-203.*) Altruism, a mature ego defense mechanism, is described as the use of constructive service to others in order to vicariously gratify one's own needs. It may include a form of benign and constructive reaction formation. Sublimation (the achieving of impulse gratification by altering the originally objectionable goal with a more acceptable one) and asceticism (obtaining gratification from renunciation of "base" pleasures) are also mature ego defenses. Reaction formation, described as the transformation of an unconscious, objectionable thought or impulse into its opposite, is a neurotic defense. Idealization refers to perception of others or oneself as totally good at the expense of a more realistic, ambivalent representation. Extremes of idealization and devaluation characterize the defense mechanism known as splitting.

310. The answer is a. (*Kaplan and Sadock, pp 953-958.*) Habit reversal training is used to eliminate dysfunctional habits such as nail biting, tics, and hair pulling. The patient is taught to recognize the triggering stimuli and the behaviors present at the very beginning of the dysfunctional habit (eg, touching the face for hair pulling). Patients are then instructed to perform an action incompatible with the habit whenever they become aware that they are on the verge of pulling their hair or biting their nails. Fist clenching is used as a competitive maneuver in both nail biting and hair pulling. Afterward, the patient is encouraged to engage in a reparatory behavior (brushing the hair or filing the nails) to remove the stimulus that may trigger future events.

311. The answer is b. (*Kaplan and Sadock, pp 202-203.*) Isolation of affect, a neurotic defense, refers to the splitting off of the affective component (usually unpleasant or unacceptable) from an idea or thought. Projection is a primitive, narcissistic defense characterized by the transposition of unacceptable feelings and ideas onto others. In projective identification, after projecting his or her own feelings and impulses onto another person, the individual acts in such a way that the other person feels compelled to act out such feelings (eg, a patient avoids becoming conscious of his anger by projecting it onto another person, then acts in a way that triggers the other person's angry feelings).

312. The answer is a. (*Kaplan and Sadock, pp 202-203.*) Acting out is behavior that is employed by the patient as a method for getting rid of unwanted emotions that are generated by the therapy process. In this case, the patient, on the verge of becoming consciously aware of his anger toward women, tries to "drown" these feelings with alcohol. Other forms of acting out include coming late to therapy sessions or missing them altogether, calling the therapist in the middle of the night, or making suicidal threats or gestures. The therapist needs to confront the patient about acting out. In this case the therapist might say, "I think you are going to the bar and drinking to excess because you are trying to numb yourself to the negative emotions that you are beginning to experience in our therapy together."

313. The answer is a. (*Ebert et al, pp 534-535.*) Since compulsive behaviors rapidly neutralize the anxiety created by obsessional thoughts, in the treatment of OCD, response prevention needs to be coupled with exposure to the feared stimulus for the exposure to be effective. Anxiety rapidly rises when the patient is prevented from performing the neutralizing compulsive behavior (eg, washing hands after touching a contaminated object), but subsequently it declines (extinction). Extinction refers to the progressive disappearance of a behavior or a symptom (in this case, anxiety) when the expected consequence does not happen (getting sick because of contamination). Desensitization refers to a gradual, graded, exposure of a patient to a feared stimulus (flying, heights, spiders, etc) coupled with relaxation training. The anxiety is inhibited by the relaxed state, a process called reciprocal inhibition.

Mood Disorders

Questions

Questions 314 and 315

314. A 30-year-old woman presents to the psychiatrist with a 2-month history of difficulty in concentrating, irritability, and depression. She has never had these symptoms before. Three months prior to her visit to the psychiatrist, the patient noted that she had experienced a short-lived flu-like illness with a rash on her calf, but has noted no other symptoms since then until the mood symptoms began. Her physical examination was within normal limits. Which of the following is the most likely diagnosis?

a. Neurosyphilis
b. Chronic meningitis
c. Lyme disease
d. Creutzfeldt-Jakob disease
e. Prion disease

315. Which of the following medications should be used to treat the patient above?

a. Penicillin
b. Antiviral medication
c. Amphotericin B
d. Doxycycline
e. Prozac for depressed mood (ie, treat the depressed mood only)

316. A 37-year-old woman comes to the physician with a chief complaint of a depressed mood. The patient states she has anhedonia, anergia, a 10-lb weight loss in the last 3 weeks, and states she "just doesn't care about anything anymore." She also admits to suicidal ideation without intent or plan. The patient is started on an SSRI. After 1 week of the medication, no improvement is seen and the dosage is raised to the maximum recommended level. Assuming there is no improvement shown, for how many weeks should this new dosage be maintained before determining that the drug trial is unsuccessful?

a. 1 to 2 weeks
b. 4 to 5 weeks
c. 8 to 9 weeks
d. 12 to 13 weeks
e. 16 or more weeks

317. A 25-year-old man comes to the psychiatrist with a chief complaint of depressed mood for 1 month. His mother, to whom he was very close, died 1 month ago, and since that time he has felt sad and been very tearful. He has difficulty concentrating, has lost 3 lb, and is not sleeping soundly through the night. Which of the following is the most likely diagnosis?

a. Major depression
b. Dysthymia
c. Posttraumatic stress disorder
d. Adjustment disorder
e. Uncomplicated bereavement

318. A 32-year-old woman is brought to the emergency room by the police after she was found standing in the middle of a busy highway, naked, commanding the traffic to stop. In the emergency room she is agitated and restless, with pressured speech and an affect that alternates between euphoric and irritable. The resident on call decides to start the patient above on a medication to control this disease. The patient refuses the medication, stating that she has taken it in the past and it causes her to be constantly thirsty, break out in pimples, and make her food taste funny. Which of the following medications is being discussed?

a. Valproic acid
b. Haloperidol
c. Carbamazepine
d. Lithium
e. Sertraline

319. A 30-year-old man comes to the psychiatrist for the evaluation of a depressed mood. He states that at least since his mid-20s he has felt depressed. He notes poor self-esteem and low energy, and feels hopeless about his situation, though he denies suicidal ideation. He states he does not use drugs or alcohol, and has no medical problems. His last physical examination by his physician 1 month ago was entirely normal. Which of the following treatment options should be tried first?

a. ECT
b. Hospitalization
c. Psychoanalysis
d. Venlafaxine
e. Amoxapine

320. A 26-year-old man comes to the physician with the chief complaint of a depressed mood for the past 5 weeks. He has been feeling down, with decreased concentration, energy, and interest in his usual hobbies. Six weeks prior to this office visit, he had been to the emergency room for an acute asthma attack and was started on prednisone. Which of the following is the most likely diagnosis?

a. Mood disorder secondary to a general medical condition
b. Substance-induced mood disorder
c. Major depression
d. Adjustment disorder
e. Dysthymia

321. What percentage of new mothers is believed to experience postpartum blues?

a. <1%
b. 10%
c. 20%
d. 50%
e. 90%

322. How long after a stroke is a patient at a higher risk for developing a depressive disorder?

a. 2 weeks
b. 2 months
c. 6 months
d. 1 year
e. 2 years

323. A 22-year-old college student calls his psychiatrist because for the past week, after cramming hard for finals, his thoughts have been racing and he is irritable. The psychiatrist notes that the patient's speech is pressured as well. The patient has been stable for the past 6 months on 500 mg of valproate twice a day, and a blood level is in the therapeutic range. Which of the following is the most appropriate first step in the management of this patient's symptoms?

a. Hospitalize the patient.
b. Increase the valproate by 500 mg/day.
c. Prescribe clonazepam 1 mg qhs.
d. Start haloperidol 5 mg qd.
e. Tell the patient to begin psychotherapy one time per week.

324. A 24-year-old woman, 5 days after delivery of a normal, full-term infant, is brought to the obstetrician because she is so tearful. She states that her mood is quite labile, often changing within minutes. She has trouble sleeping, both falling asleep and awakening early. She notes anhedonia, stating she doesn't enjoy "much of anything" right now. Which of this patient's symptoms point preferentially to a postpartum depression as opposed to postpartum blues?

a. Time—that is, 5 days post delivery
b. Tearfulness
c. Labile mood
d. Insomnia
e. Anhedonia

325. A 28-year-old woman sees her physician with the chief complaint of a depressed mood for the past 4 weeks, since just after the Christmas season. She also notes that she is sleeping more than usual—up to 14 hours per night—but does not feel rested and that she feels tired and fatigued all the time. She has gained 14 lb in the last month, something that she is very unhappy about, but she says that she seems to have such a craving for sweets that the weight gain seemed inevitable. Thyroid function tests are within normal limits. Which of the following is the most likely diagnosis?

a. Mood disorder secondary to a general medical condition
b. Substance-induced mood disorder
c. Cyclothymia
d. Seasonal affective disorder
e. Dysthymic disorder

326. A 38-year-old woman with bipolar disorder has been stable on lithium for the past 2 years. She comes to her psychiatrist's office in tears after a 2-week history of a depressed mood, poor concentration, loss of appetite, and passive suicidal ideation. Which of the following is the most appropriate next step in the management of this patient?

a. Start the patient on a second mood stabilizer.
b. Start the patient on a long-acting benzodiazepine.
c. Stop the lithium and start an antidepressant.
d. Start an antidepressant and continue the lithium.
e. Stop the lithium and start an antipsychotic.

327. A 27-year-old woman has been feeling blue for the past 2 weeks. She has little energy and has trouble concentrating. She states that 6 weeks ago she had been feeling very good, with lots of energy and no need for sleep. She says that this pattern has been occurring for at least the past 3 years, though the episodes have never been so severe that she couldn't work. Which of the following is the most likely diagnosis?

a. Borderline personality disorder
b. Seasonal affective disorder
c. Cyclothymic disorder
d. Major depression, recurrent
e. Bipolar disorder, depressed

328. A 19-year-old woman comes to the psychiatrist for a history of anger and irritability, which occurs once monthly on average. During this time the patient also reports feeling anxious and "about to explode," which alternates rapidly with crying spells and angry outbursts. The patient notes during this time she can't concentrate and sleeps much more than she usually needs to do. During the several days these symptoms last, the patient must skip most of her classes because she cannot function. Which of the following is the most likely diagnosis?

a. Adjustment disorder with depressed mood
b. Major depression
c. Premenstrual dysphoric disorder
d. Dysthymic disorder
e. Depressive personality disorder

329. A 42-year-old woman sees her physician because she has been depressed for the past 4 months. She also notes that she has gained 20 lb without trying to. She notes that she does not take pleasure in the activities that she once enjoyed and seems fatigued most of the time. These symptoms have caused the patient to withdraw from many of the social functions that she once enjoyed. The physician diagnoses the patient with hypothyroidism and starts her on thyroid supplementation. Six weeks later, the patient's thyroid hormone levels have normalized, but she still reports feeling depressed. Which of the following is the most appropriate next step in the management of this patient?

a. Recommend that the patient begin psychotherapy.
b. Increase the patient's thyroid supplementation.
c. Start the patient on an antidepressant medication.
d. Tell the patient that she should wait another 6 weeks, during which time her mood will improve.
e. Take a substance abuse history from the patient.

330. A 64-year-old man is admitted to the psychiatric unit after an unsuccessful suicide attempt. Following admission, he attempts to cut his wrists three times in the next 24 hours and refuses to eat or drink anything. He is scheduled to have electroconvulsive therapy (ECT) because he is so severely depressed that an antidepressant is deemed too slow acting. Which of the following side effects should the patient be informed is most common after ECT?

a. Headache
b. Palpitations
c. Deep venous thromboses
d. Interictal confusion
e. Worsening of the suicidal ideation

331. A 14-year-old boy is brought to the psychiatrist because for the past 15 months he has been irritable and depressed almost constantly. The boy notes that he has difficulty concentrating, and he has lost 5 lb during that time period without trying. He states that he feels as if he has always been depressed, and he feels hopeless about ever feeling better. He denies suicidal ideation or hallucinations. He is sleeping well and doing well in school, though his teachers have noticed that he does not seem to be able to concentrate as well as he had previously. Which of the following is the most likely diagnosis?

a. Major depression
b. Dysthymic disorder
c. Mood disorder secondary to a general medical condition
d. Normal adolescence
e. Cyclothymia

332. A 29-year-old man is brought to the hospital because he was found running around on the streets with no shoes on in the middle of winter, screaming to everyone that he was going to be elected president. Upon admission to the hospital, he was stabilized on olanzapine and lithium and then discharged home. Assuming the patient is maintained on the olanzapine and the lithium, which of the following tests should be performed at least once per year?

a. MRI of the brain
b. Liver function tests
c. Creatinine level
d. Rectal examination to look for the presence of blood in the stool
e. ECG

333. A 45-year-old woman comes to her physician for help with her insomnia. She states "ever since my husband died, I just can't sleep." The patient states her 57-year-old husband died suddenly of a heart attack 9 weeks ago. Since that time, the patient has had a very depressed mood, has been crying, has lost interest in activities, is fatigued, and has insomnia. Which of the following symptoms, if present, should make the physician think this patient has a major depression instead of bereavement?

a. The patient feels that she would be better off dead without her husband.
b. The patient has marked functional impairment.
c. The patient has lots of guilt about not recognizing that the chest pain her husband was having was the start of a heart attack.
d. The patient has mild psychomotor retardation.
e. The patient reports hearing the voice of her dead husband calling her name twice.

334. A 10-year-old boy is brought to the psychiatrist by his mother. She states that for the past 2 months he has been increasingly irritable, withdrawn, and apathetic. He has been refusing to do his homework, and his grades have dropped. Which of the following is the best next step in management?

a. The child should be hospitalized.
b. The child should be started in supportive psychotherapy.
c. The mother should be warned that the child will likely turn out to be bipolar (67% chance).
d. The child should receive an antidepressant medication.
e. The child should receive lithium and an antidepressant.

335. A 35-year-old woman is seeing a psychiatrist for treatment of her major depression. After 4 weeks on fluoxetine at 40 mg/day, her psychiatrist decides to try augmentation. Which of the following is the most appropriate medication?

a. Lithium
b. Sertraline
c. An MAO inhibitor
d. Clonazepam
e. Haloperidol

336. Which of the following is a contraindication for ECT?

a. Space-occupying lesion in the brain
b. Pregnancy
c. Hypertension
d. Seizure disorder
e. Status post–myocardial infarction 6 months earlier

337. A middle-aged woman presents with a variety of cognitive and somatic symptoms, fatigue, and memory loss. She denies feeling sad, but her family physician is aware of this patient's lifelong inability to identify and express feelings. He suspects she is depressed. Which of the following results is most likely to confirm a diagnosis of depression?

a. Reduced metabolic activity and blood flow in both frontal lobes on PET scan
b. Diffuse cortical atrophy on CAT scan
c. Atrophy of the caudate on MRI
d. Prolonged REM sleep latency in a sleep study
e. Subcortical infarcts on MRI

338. A 32-year-old man is being treated for a severe major depression. Which of the following symptoms, if present, is one of the most accurate indicators of long-term suicidal risk?

a. Revenge fantasies
b. Presence of rage in the patient
c. Hopelessness
d. Presence of guilt
e. Presence of a need for punishment in patient

Questions 339 to 342

Match each patient's symptoms with the most appropriate diagnosis. Each lettered option may be used once, more than once, or not at all.

a. Atypical depression
b. Double depression
c. Cyclothymic disorder
d. Melancholic depression
e. Schizoaffective disorder
f. Seasonal affective disorder

339. An elderly man has been profoundly depressed for several weeks. He cries easily and is intensely preoccupied with trivial episodes from his past, which he considers unforgivable sins. This patient awakens every morning at 3 AM and cannot go back to sleep. Anything his family has tried to cheer him up has failed. He has completely lost his appetite and appears gaunt and emaciated.

340. A young woman, who has felt mildly unhappy and dissatisfied with herself for most of her life has been severely depressed, irritable, and anhedonic for 3 weeks.

341. For the past 6 weeks, a middle-aged woman's mood has been mostly depressed, but she cheers up briefly when her grandchildren visit or in coincidence with other pleasant events. She is consistently less depressed in the morning than at night. When her children fail to call on the phone to inquire about her health, her mood deteriorates even more. She sleeps 14 hours every night and has gained 24 lb.

342. Since he moved to Maine from his native Florida 3 years earlier, a college student has had great difficulty preparing for the winter-term courses. He starts craving for sweets and feeling sluggish, fatigued, and irritable in late October. These symptoms worsen gradually during the following months, and by February he has consistently gained several pounds. His mood and energy level start improving in March, and by May he is back to baseline.

Mood Disorders

Answers

314 and 315. The answers are 314-c, 315-d. (*Kaplan and Sadock, p 366.*) Lyme disease is characterized by a bull's-eye rash at the site of the tick bite, followed by a flu-like illness which is often short-lived and may go unnoticed. Problems with cognitive functioning and mood changes may be the first complaints seen. These include problems concentrating, irritability, fatigue, and a depressed mood. Treatment consists of a 2- to 3-week course of doxycycline, which is curative about 90% of the time. If the disease is left untreated, 60% of patients will develop a chronic condition.

316. The answer is b. (*Kaplan and Sadock, pp 530-531, 557.*) Elevated HPA levels are a hallmark of stress in mammals, and provide a clear link between the biology of stress and depression. Lymphocytic proliferation in response to mitogens is decreased in depression. Both core body temperature and phasic rapid eye movement (REM) sleep are increased in those with depression. A widely replicated finding on PET scans in patients with depression is a decreased anterior brain metabolism. There are numerous other physiologic changes associated with depressions as well. The most common clinical mistake made when treating a patient with a major depression is to put the patient on a dose of an antidepressant that is too low, or is used for too short a time. Doses of antidepressants should generally be raised to their maximal doses and kept there for 4 to 5 weeks before a drug trial is considered unsuccessful. However, if a patient is doing well on a low dose of an antidepressant, that dosage should not be raised unless clinical improvement stops before the patient has reached his maximum benefit from the drug.

317. The answer is e. (*Kaplan and Sadock, pp 64-68.*) The loss of a loved one is often accompanied by symptoms reminiscent of major depression, such as sadness, weepiness, insomnia, reduced appetite, and weight loss. When these symptoms do not persist beyond 2 months after the loss, they are considered a normal manifestation of bereavement. A diagnosis of major depression in these circumstances requires the presence of marked functional impairment, morbid preoccupations with unrealistic guilt or worthlessness, suicidal ideation, marked psychomotor retardation, and psychotic symptoms, on top of the symptoms listed in the first sentence above. A diagnosis of adjustment disorder with depressed mood would not normally be given to someone when the "adjustment" is to the recent death of a loved one—instead, bereavement is the diagnosis given (complicated or uncomplicated).

318. The answer is d. (*Kaplan and Sadock, pp 560-562.*) Lithium is still the treatment of choice for acute mania and maintenance, although anticonvulsants such as valproate and carbamazepine have been proven effective. Newer anticonvulsants, such as gabapentin, topiramate, and lamotrigine, have also proved to have mood-stabilizing properties, although these medications have not been extensively studied yet. Weight gain, metallic taste, acne, hypothyroidism, and polyuria are common complaints with long-term lithium treatment.

319. The answer is d. (*Kaplan and Sadock, pp 563-566.*) This patient has a dysthymic disorder. While many clinicians do not believe that these disorders should be treated pharmacologically, there are a number of studies that show positive responses to antidepressants with these patients. Venlafaxine and bupropion are generally believed to be the treatments of choice for dysthymic disorder, though there is a subgroup of patients that will respond to the MAOIs as well.

320. The answer is b. (*Kaplan and Sadock, pp 573-577.*) According to *DSM-IV* criteria, patients developing a mood disorder after using a substance (either illicit or prescribed) are diagnosed with a substance-induced mood disorder. The diagnosis of major depression cannot be made in the presence of either substance use or a general medical condition that might be the cause of the mood disorder. Prednisone is a common culprit in causing mood disorders ranging from depression to mania to psychosis.

321. The answer is d. (*Kaplan and Sadock, p 865.*) Postpartum blues is extremely common in women who give birth, with upwards of 30% to 75% of women experiencing it in the 3 to 5 days after delivery. There is no association of mood disorders with this syndrome, and suicidal thoughts are not present. The blues typically last days to weeks, then remit spontaneously without treatment.

322. The answer is e. (*Kaplan and Sadock, p 1086.*) Studies of the course and prognosis of poststroke depression indicate that the high-risk period can last up to 2 years. The presence of depression is associated with an eightfold increase in mortality risk.

323. The answer is c. (*Kaplan and Sadock, p 127.*) Sleep deprivation has an antidepressant effect in depressed patients and may trigger a manic episode in bipolar patients. The patient is not ill enough to require hospitalization. The use of a long-acting benzodiazepine will allow the patient to return to a normal sleep pattern and generally will abort the manic episode.

324. The answer is e. (*Kaplan and Sadock, p 865.*) All of the symptoms that this patient is experiencing except one are congruent with the postpartum blues. These symptoms may last several days, and are thought to be secondary to the combination of large hormonal shifts and the awareness of increased responsibility for a new human being. Anhedonia is not seen in postpartum blues, but is common in postpartum depressions.

325. The answer is d. (*Moore and Jefferson, pp 136, 140.*) Patients with seasonal affective disorder typically present in just the way this patient has. Patients usually exhibit typical signs and symptoms seasonally, most often during the winter, with symptoms remitting in the spring. Hypersomnia and hyperphagia (atypical signs of a depression) are classically seen with this disorder. Light therapy and serotonergic agents (typically SSRIs) are the treatments of choice for this disorder.

326. The answer is d. (*Kaplan and Sadock, p 561.*) Since lithium and other mood stabilizers are more effective in the prevention of manic episodes than in the prevention of depression, antidepressants are used as an adjunctive treatment when depressive episodes develop during maintenance with a mood stabilizer. Since the incidence of antidepressant-induced mania is high (up to 30%), and since antidepressant treatment may cause rapid cycling, the antidepressant should be tapered and discontinued as soon as the depressive symptoms remit. Among the antidepressants in common use, bupropion is considered to carry a slightly lower risk of triggering mania.

327. The answer is c. (*Kaplan and Sadock, pp 566-567.*) Cyclothymic disorder is characterized by recurrent periods of mild depression alternating with periods of hypomania. This pattern must be present for at least 2 years

(1 year for children and adolescents) before the diagnosis can be made. During these 2 years, the symptom-free intervals should not be longer than 2 months. Cyclothymic disorder usually starts during adolescence or early adulthood and tends to have a chronic course. The marked shifts in mood of cyclothymic disorder can be confused with the affective instability of borderline personality disorder or may suggest a substance abuse problem.

328. The answer is c. (*Kaplan and Sadock, p 867.*) Premenstrual dysphoric disorder is an illness which is triggered by the changing levels of hormones that occur during a menstrual cycle. It occurs approximately 1 week before the onset of menses and is characterized by headaches, anxiety, depression, irritability, and emotional lability. Other symptoms include edema, weight gain, and breast pain. Approximately 5% of women suffer from this disorder. Some patients respond to short courses of SSRIs, in addition to symptomatic treatment with analgesics and diuretics.

329. The answer is c. (*Moore and Jefferson, pp 293-295.*) This patient is likely suffering from a mood disorder secondary to a general medical condition, characterized by a depressed mood and loss of interest in activities she usually enjoyed. It is interesting to note that many of these mood disorders, especially those caused by an endocrine disorder, persist even after the underlying medical condition has been treated. In that case (and in the case described in this question), the physician should begin the patient on antidepressant medication.

330. The answer is a. (*Moore and Jefferson, pp 518-521.*) The most common complaints after ECT include headaches, nausea, and muscle soreness. Memory impairment (both retrograde and anterograde) does occur but less frequently, and interictal confusion is quite uncommon. Likewise, cardiovascular changes do occur, but they are rare and happen mostly in the immediate postictal period or during the seizure itself.

331. The answer is b. (*Moore and Jefferson, pp 142-143.*) This patient is suffering from a dysthymic disorder, characterized by an irritable or depressed mood for at least 1 year. (This patient is an adolescent—if he were an adult, the time requirement for the diagnosis of dysthymic would be 2 years.) The patient complains of difficulty concentrating and has had some weight loss. He also feels hopeless about ever not feeling depressed. However, he has no suicidal ideation or psychotic symptoms and no other vegetative symptoms. He is still doing well in school, a clue that the depression is probably not severe enough to rate a diagnosis of major depression, especially when combined with the length of time that this patient has been depressed and irritable.

332. The answer is c. *(Jacobson and Jacobson, p 263.)* This patient, likely suffering from bipolar disorder, mania, is being maintained on lithium and an antipsychotic. Patients on lithium, at minimum, should be monitored for the following: plasma lithium level (once every month or two until the patient is stable, and then less frequently if he or she is reliable), thyroid function tests, creatinine, and urinalysis. ECGs are part of the list of optional recommendations for patients on lithium but are generally reserved for patients over the age of 50. There are no standard blood tests or other examinations to monitor use of olanzapine.

333. The answer is b. *(Kaplan and Sadock, p 889.)* This patient is suffering from bereavement, which normally begins immediately after, or within a short time of the death of a loved one. There are certain symptoms that are not characteristic of a "normal" grief reaction and may help in the differentiation of bereavement from a major depression. These include (1) guilt about things other than actions taken or not taken by the survivor at the time of the loved one's death, (2) thoughts of death other than the survivor feeling he/she would be better off dead without the loved one, (3) a morbid preoccupation with worthlessness, (4) marked psychomotor retardation, (5) marked and prolonged functional impairment, and (6) hallucinations other than the survivor believing he/she can hear the voice or see the loved one.

334. The answer is d. *(Kaplan and Sadock, pp 1260-1262.)* Major depression is not a rare occurrence in children. Prevalence rates are 0.3% in preschoolers, 0.4% to 3% in school-age children, and 0.4% to 4.6% in adolescents. Making a correct diagnosis is complicated by the fact that the presentation of juvenile depression often differs from the adult presentation. Depressed preschoolers tend to be irritable, aggressive, withdrawn, or clingy instead of sad. In school-age children, the main manifestation of depression may be a significant loss of interest in friends and school. By adolescence, presenting symptoms of depression become more similar to those of adults. Psychotic symptoms are common in depressed children, most commonly one voice that makes depreciative comments and mood-congruent delusional ideations. Up to one-third of children diagnosed with major depression receive a diagnosis of bipolar disorder later in life. This evolution is more likely when the depressive episode has an abrupt onset and is accompanied by psychotic symptoms. Childhood depression can be treated pharmacologically, but child response to medication differs from adult response. SSRIs have been proven effective in preschoolers and school-age children; tricyclic antidepressants (TCAs) have not. There are insufficient data about the efficacy of newer antidepressants such as nefazodone, venlafaxine, bupropion, and mirtazapine. The response of older adolescents to antidepressants is equivalent to the adult response. Supportive psychotherapy alone is likely to be ineffective in treatment of a childhood major depression.

335. The answer is a. (*Kaplan and Sadock, pp 1056-1058.*) Lithium has been proven effective when added to an antidepressant in the treatment of refractory depression. More than one mechanism of action is probably involved, although lithium's ability to increase the presynaptic release of serotonin is the best understood. Other augmentation strategies include the use of thyroid hormones, stimulants, estrogens, and light therapy. The combination of two SSRIs (in this case, fluoxetine and sertraline) or of an MAOI and an SSRI is not recommended because of the risk of precipitating a serotonin syndrome.

336. The answer is a. (*Kaplan and Sadock, pp 1117-1120.*) ECT is a safe procedure with very few contraindications (myocardial infarcts within the past 4 weeks, increased intracranial pressure, aneurysms, bleeding disorders, and any condition that disrupts the blood-brain barrier).

337. The answer is a. (*Kaplan and Sadock, pp 81-85.*) Positron emission tomography (PET) scan has consistently demonstrated a decrease in blood flow and metabolism in the frontal lobe of depressed patients. Most studies have found bilateral rather than unilateral deficits and equivalent decreases in several types of depression (unipolar, bipolar, associated with OCD). Cortical atrophy and subcortical infarcts are associated, respectively, with Alzheimer disease and multi-infarct dementia. Atrophy of the caudate is characteristic of Huntington disease. In major depression, the REM sleep latency (the period of time between falling asleep and the first period of REM sleep) is shortened, not prolonged.

338. The answer is c. *(Kaplan and Sadock, p 900.)* A study by Beck showed that hopelessness is one of the most accurate indicators of long-term suicidal risk. No one specific psychodynamic or personality structure is associated with higher risks of suicide. Revenge fantasies, overwhelming affects such as guilt or rage, or the patient's unconscious wish for punishment can all precipitate a suicide attempt.

339 to 342. The answers are 339-d, 340-b, 341-a, 342-f. *(Kaplan and Sadock, pp 527-578.)* Melancholic depression, a variant of major depressive disorder, is characterized by loss of pleasure in all activities (anhedonia), lack of reactivity (nothing can make the patient feel better), intense guilt, significant weight loss, early morning awakening, and marked psychomotor retardation. TCAs have been considered to be more effective than other antidepressants in the treatment of melancholic depression.

Double depression is diagnosed when a major depressive episode develops in a patient with dysthymic disorder. Between 68% and 90% of patients with dysthymic disorder experience at least one episode of major depression during their lives. Compared with patients who are euthymic between depressive episodes, dysthymic patients with superimposed major depression experience a higher risk for suicide, more severe depressive symptoms, more psychosocial impairment, and more treatment resistance.

Atypical depression, another variant of major depressive disorder, is characterized by mood reactivity (pleasurable events may temporarily improve the mood), self-pity, excessive sensitivity to rejection, reversed diurnal mood fluctuations (patients feel better in the morning), and reversed vegetative symptoms (increased appetite and increased sleep). Approximately 15% of patients with depression have atypical features. MAOIs are considered to be more effective than other classes of antidepressants in atypical depression.

Seasonal affective disorder is characterized by a regular temporal relationship between the appearance of symptoms of depression or mania and a particular time of the year. Depression characteristically starts in the fall and resolves spontaneously in spring, with a mean duration of 5 to 6 months. Characteristic symptoms include irritability, increased appetite with carbohydrate craving, increased sleep, and increased weight. The shortening of the day is the precipitant for seasonal depression. Manic episodes are associated with increased length of daylight and, consequently, with the summer months.

Anxiety, Somatoform, and Dissociative Disorders

Questions

343. A 23-year-old woman arrives at the emergency room complaining that, out of the blue, she had been seized by an overwhelming fear associated with shortness of breath and a pounding heart. These symptoms lasted for approximately 20 minutes, and while she was experiencing them, she feared that she was dying or going crazy. The patient has had four similar episodes during the past month, and she has been worrying that they will continue to recur. Which of the following is the most likely diagnosis?

a. Acute psychotic episode
b. Hypochondriasis
c. Panic disorder
d. Generalized anxiety disorder
e. Posttraumatic stress disorder

344. A middle-aged man is chronically preoccupied with his health. For many years he feared that his irregular bowel functions meant he had cancer. Now he is very worried about having a serious heart disease, despite his physician's assurance that the occasional "extra beats" he detects when he checks his pulse are completely benign. Which of the following is the most likely diagnosis?

a. Somatization disorder
b. Hypochondriasis
c. Delusional disorder
d. Pain disorder
e. Conversion disorder

Questions 345 to 347

Match the following classical presentations with its diagnosis. Each lettered option may be used once, more than once, or not at all.

a. Somatization disorder
b. Conversion disorder
c. Hypochondriasis
d. Body dysmorphic disorder
e. Pain disorder

345. A 20-year-old woman comes to her primary care doctor with multiple symptoms which are present across several organ systems. She has seen five doctors in the past 3 months, and has had six surgeries since the age of 18.

346. A 17-year-old girl presents to a physician complaining that her face is "out of proportion" and that she looks like "Mr Hyde—like a monster." On examination, the girl is a pleasant-looking young woman with no facial deformities of any kind.

347. A 45-year-old woman presents to her physician with a chief complaint of a severe headache that is increasing in severity over the past 3 weeks. The patient states that 1 month ago she was in an auto accident and was diagnosed with a concussion. The patient states that the headache has been increasing since then and she is completely unable to work. The MRI of her head is normal.

348. A 28-year-old taxi driver is chronically consumed by fears of having accidentally run over a pedestrian. Although he tries to convince himself that his worries are silly, his anxiety continues to mount until he drives back to the scene of the "accident" and proves to himself that nobody lies hurt in the street. This behavior best exemplifies which of the following?

a. A compulsion secondary to an obsession
b. An obsession triggered by a compulsion
c. A delusional ideation
d. A typical manifestation of obsessive-compulsive personality disorder
e. A phobia

349. A young woman, who has a very limited memory of her childhood years but knows that she was removed from her parents because of their abuse and neglect, frequently cannot account for hours or even days of her life. She hears voices that alternately plead, reprimand, or simply comment on what she is doing. Occasionally, she does not remember how and when she arrived at a specific location. She finds clothes she does not like in her closet, and she does not remember having bought them. Her friends are puzzled because sometimes she acts in a childish, dependent way and at other times becomes uncharacteristically aggressive and controlling. These symptoms are most commonly seen in which of the following disorders?

a. Dissociative amnesia
b. Depersonalization disorder
c. Korsakoff dementia
d. Dissociative identity disorder
e. Schizophrenia

Questions 350 and 351

350. A 34-year-old secretary climbs 12 flights of stairs every day to reach her office because she is terrified by the thought of being trapped in the elevator. She has never had any traumatic event occur in an elevator; nonetheless, she has been terrified of them since childhood. Which of the following is the most likely diagnosis?

a. Social phobia
b. Performance anxiety
c. Generalized anxiety disorder
d. Specific phobia
e. Agoraphobia

351. Which of the following is the treatment of choice for the patient described in the previous vignette?

a. Imipramine
b. Clonazepam
c. Propanolol
d. Exposure therapy
e. Psychoanalysis

352. A 26-year-old woman comes to the psychiatrist with a 1-month history of severe anxiety. The patient states that 1 month ago she was a "normal, laid-back person." Since that time she rates her anxiety an 8 on a scale of 1 to 10, and also notes she is afraid to leave the house unless she checks that the door is locked at least five times. Which of the following medical conditions could commonly cause this kind of symptom presentation?

a. Hyperglycemia
b. Crohn disease
c. Hyperparathyroidism
d. Fibromyalgia
e. Peptic ulcer disease

353. A 28-year-old business executive sees her physician because she is having difficulty in her new position, because it requires her to do frequent public speaking. She states that she is terrified she will do or say something that will cause her extreme embarrassment. The patient says that when she must speak in public, she becomes extremely anxious and her heart beats uncontrollably. Other than in these performance situations, she does not find herself anxious generally. Based on this clinical picture, which of the following medications is likely to be the best choice for this patient?

a. Fluoxetine daily
b. Propranolol prn
c. Bupropion daily
d. Olanzepine daily
e. Clonazepam prn

Questions 354 to 356

Match each patient's symptoms with the most likely diagnosis. Each lettered option may be used once, more than once, or not at all.

a. Agoraphobia
b. Panic disorder
c. Obsessive-compulsive disorder
d. Social phobia
e. Adjustment disorder
f. Specific phobia
g. Acute stress disorder

354. A 45-year-old policeman who has demonstrated great courage on more than one occasion while on duty is terrified of needles.

355. For several months, a 32-year-old housewife has been unable to leave her house unaccompanied. When she tries to go out alone, she is overwhelmed by anxiety and fears that something terrible will happen to her and nobody will be there to help.

356. A 17-year-old girl blushes, stammers, and feels completely foolish when one of her classmates or a teacher asks her a question. She sits at the back of the class hoping not to be noticed because she is convinced that the other students think she is unattractive and stupid.

Questions 357 to 361

Match each patient's symptoms with the most likely diagnosis. Each lettered option may be used once, more than once, or not at all.
a. Somatization disorder
b. Specific phobia
c. Dissociative identity disorder
d. Obsessive-compulsive disorder
e. Dissociative fugue
f. Posttraumatic stress disorder
g. Body dysmorphic disorder
h. Dysthymia

357. Two years after she was saved from her burning house, a 32-year-old woman continues to be distressed by recurrent dreams and intrusive thoughts about the event.

358. A 20-year-old student is very distressed by a small deviation of his nasal septum. He is convinced that this minor imperfection is disfiguring, although others barely notice it.

359. A nun is found in a distant city working in a cabaret. She is unable to remember anything about her previous life.

360. A 35-year-old woman is often late to work because she must shower and dress in a very particular order or else she becomes increasingly anxious.

361. For the past 3 years, a 24-year-old college student has suffered from chronic headaches, fatigue, shortness of breath, dizziness, ringing ears, and constipation. He is incensed when his primary physician recommends a psychiatric evaluation because no organic cause for his symptoms could be found.

Questions 362 to 364

Match the following patients' symptoms with the most appropriate pharmacological treatment. Each lettered option may be used once, more than once, or not at all.

a. Antipsychotic
b. Antianxiety agent (non-benzodiazepine)
c. Tricyclic antidepressant
d. Mood stabilizer
e. SSRI
f. Beta-blocker

362. A woman washes her hands hundreds of times a day out of a fear of contamination. She cannot stop herself, although her hands are raw and chafed.

363. A middle-aged bank teller with a past history of alcohol abuse, who describes himself as a chronic worrier, has been promoted to a position with increased responsibilities. Since the promotion, he has been constantly worrying about his job. He fears his superiors have made a mistake and they will soon realize he is not the right person for that position. He ruminates about unlikely future catastrophes, such as not being able to pay his bills and having to declare bankruptcy if he is fired. He has trouble falling asleep at night and suffers from acid indigestion.

364. A talented 21-year-old violinist's musical career is in jeopardy because he becomes acutely anxious whenever he is asked to play in front of an audience.

365. A 24-year-old woman comes to the psychiatrist with a 2-month history of short episodes of "feeling like I am going to die." During these episodes, she also notes feelings of dizziness and nausea, along with a feeling of choking. She describes these episodes as very frightening and she is terrified of having another. She denies substance use or any medical problems. Which of the following treatment regimens should be started?

a. Imipramine
b. Fluoxetine
c. Phenelzine
d. Paroxetine and alprazolam
e. Buspirone and citalopram

Anxiety, Somatoform, and Dissociative Disorders

Answers

343. The answer is c. *(Jacobson and Jacobson, p 5.)* This patient displays typical symptoms of recurrent panic attacks. Panic attacks can occur under a wide variety of psychiatric and medical conditions. The patient is diagnosed with panic disorder when there are recurrent episodes of panic and there is at least 1 month of persistent concern, worry, or behavioral change associated with the attacks. The attacks are not because of the direct effect of medical illness, medications, or substance abuse and are not better accounted for by another psychiatric disorder. While anxiety can be intense in generalized anxiety disorder, major depression, acute psychosis, and hypochondriasis, it does not have the typical presentation (ie, a discrete episode or panic attack) described in this question.

344. The answer is b. *(Moore and Jefferson, pp 181-183.)* Hypochondriasis is characterized by fear of developing or having a serious disease, based on the patient's distorted interpretation of normal physical sensations or signs. The patient continues to worry even though physical examinations and diagnostic tests fail to reveal any pathological process. The fears do not have the absolute certainty of delusions. Hypochondriasis can develop in every age group, but onset is most common between 20 and 30 years of age. Both genders are equally represented, and there are no differences in prevalence based on social, educational, or marital status. The disorder tends to have a chronic, relapsing course.

345 to 347. The answers are 345-a, 346-d, 347-e. *(Kaplan and Sadock, p 635.)* Somatization disorder is characterized by a polysymptomatic presentation, with the patient presenting as someone who has been chronically sick. Females present with this disorder about 20 times more frequently than do males, and there is a 5% to 10% incidence in the primary care population. Patients have often had multiple surgeries. Patients with conversion disorder are generally young females with poor education; they typically are from rural areas and low socioeconomic class. They present acutely, usually with one symptom, but that symptom may be incompatible with known pathophysiologic mechanisms. Patients with hypochondriasis tend to be older, and men and women present with equal frequency. Patients are overconcerned with a disease, which amplifies their symptoms as a result. They are usually temporarily reassured with negative test findings, but soon find another illness to obsess about. Patients with a body dysmorphic disorder tend to be young (adolescence to age 40 at diagnosis) and are represented equally in gender. They have subjective feelings that they are ugly or have some body part that is deformed. Those with pain disorders are usually in their fourth or fifth decade of life, with women represented in the population twice as often as men. These patients have often had some precipitating event to their pain, but it continues with an intensity incompatible with known physiologic mechanisms.

348. The answer is a. *(Jacobson and Jacobson, pp 85-91.)* Recurrent obsessions and compulsions are essential features of obsessive-compulsive disorder (OCD). Obsessions are persistent thoughts or mental images that are subjectively experienced as intrusive and alien and characteristically provoke various levels of anxiety. Compulsions are repetitive acts, behaviors, or thoughts designed to counteract the anxiety elicited by the obsessions. Thus obsessions (which cause anxiety) are paired with their related compulsions (which help manage the anxiety produced). The diagnosis of obsessive-compulsive personality disorder is reserved for those patients with significant impairments in their occupational or social effectiveness. These patients are preoccupied with rules, regulations, orderliness, neatness, details, and the achievement of perfection.

349. The answer is d. *(Jacobson and Jacobson, pp 187-188.)* Losing time and memory gaps, including significant gaps in autobiographical memory, are typical symptoms of dissociative identity disorder (previously known as multiple personality disorder). Patients also report fluctuation in their skills, well-learned abilities, and habits. This is explained as a state-dependent disturbance of implicit memory. Hallucinations in all sensory modalities are common. Dramatic changes in mannerisms, tone of voice, and affect are manifestations of this disorder.

350. The answer is d. (*Jacobson and Jacobson, p 80.*) Specific phobias are characterized by an unreasonable or excessive fear of an object, an animal, or a situation (flying, being trapped in close spaces, heights, blood, spiders, etc). Since the exposure to the feared situation, animal, or object causes an immediate surge of anxiety, patients carefully avoid the phobic stimuli. The diagnosis of specific phobia requires the presence of reduced functioning and interference with social activities and relationships because of the avoidant behavior, anticipatory anxiety, and distress caused by the exposure to the feared stimulus. In social phobias and performance anxiety, patients fear social interactions (in general or limited to specific situations) and public performance (public speaking, acting, playing an instrument), respectively. In generalized anxiety disorder, the anxiety is more chronic and less intense than in a phobic disorder and is not limited to a specific situation or item. Agoraphobic patients fear places where escape may be difficult or help may not be available in case the patient has a panic attack. Agoraphobic patients are often prisoners in their own homes and depend on a companion when they need to go out.

351. The answer is d. (*Jacobson and Jacobson, p 217.*) No medication has proven to be effective in treating specific phobias. The treatment of choice for specific phobias is exposure, in vivo or using techniques of guided imagery, pairing relaxation exercises with exposure to the feared stimulus. The patient can be exposed to the feared stimulus gradually or can be asked to immediately confront the most anxiety-provoking situation (flooding).

352. The answer is c. (*Kaplan and Sadock, p 354.*) Medical conditions that can cause anxiety-related symptoms include the endocrinopathies (pheochromocytoma, hyperthyroidism, hypercortisolemic states, and hyperparathyroidism), metabolic problems (hypoxemia, hypercalcemia, and hypoglycemia) and neurologic disorders, including vascular, trauma, and degenerative types. Although mitral valve prolapse and panic attacks have long been associated, the mitral valve prolapse actually causing the panic attacks is not known.

353. The answer is b. (*Kaplan and Sadock, p 604.*) While fluoxetine and clonazepam may both be used effectively in cases of generalized social phobia, this young woman reports feeling extremely anxious only under performance situations. For control of performance anxiety, either β-adrenergic receptor antagonists (commonly atenolol or propranolol) or relatively short acting benzodiazepines (lorazepam or alprazolam) are the treatments of choice. The antipsychotic olanzepine would be an inappropriate choice in either case of generalized social phobia or social phobia related to performance anxiety.

354 to 356. The answers are 354-f, 355-a, 356-d. *(Moore and Jefferson, pp 163-167.)* Phobic disorders include agoraphobia, specific phobias, and social phobia. They are all characterized by overwhelming, persistent, and irrational fears that result in the overpowering need to avoid the object or situation that is generating the anxiety. Agoraphobia is the marked fear and avoidance of being alone in public places where rapid exit would be difficult or help would not be available. Social phobia is characterized by avoidance of situations in which one is exposed to scrutiny by others and by fears of being humiliated or embarrassed by one's actions. Specific phobias are triggered by objects (often animals), heights, or closed spaces. A large variety of objects are associated with simple phobias.

357 to 361. The answers are 357-f, 358-g, 359-e, 360-d, 361-a. *(Moore and Jefferson, pp 158-175.)* One of the most characteristic features of post-traumatic stress disorder (PTSD) is the occurrence of repeated dreams, flashbacks, and intrusive thoughts of the traumatic event. Hyperarousal, irritability, difficulties concentrating, exaggerated startle response, emotional numbing, avoidance of places and situations associated with the traumatic experience, dissociative amnesia, and a sense of foreshortened future are other symptoms displayed by patients with PTSD. In body dysmorphic disorder, a person of normal appearance is preoccupied with some imaginary physical defect. The belief is tenacious and sometimes of delusional intensity. This diagnosis should not be made when the distorted ideations are limited to the belief of being fat in anorexia nervosa or to uneasiness with one's gender characteristics in gender identity disorder. Patients with obsessive-compulsive disorder (OCD) experience persistent thoughts, impulses, or repetitive behaviors that they are unable to stop voluntarily. Obsessions and compulsions are experienced as alien and egodystonic and are the source of much distress. Somatization disorder is characterized by a history of multiple physical complaints not explained by organic factors. The diagnosis requires the presence of four pain symptoms, two gastrointestinal symptoms, one sexual symptom, and one pseudoneurological symptom over the course of the disorder. The essential feature of dissociative fugue is sudden travel away from home accompanied by temporary loss of autobiographic memory. Patients are confused about their identity and at times form new identities. Dissociative fugue may last from hours to months. During the fugue, individuals do not appear to have any psychopathology; usually they come to attention when their identity is questioned.

362 to 364. The answers are 362-e, 363-b, 364-f. (*Moore and Jefferson, pp 158-175.*) The patient who compulsively washes her hands has obsessive-compulsive disorder (OCD), and she would respond to an SSRI. Treatment of OCD symptoms may require higher dosages and longer trial periods than those recommended for depression. Before a trial is considered ineffective, the patient should have received minimum daily doses of sertraline 200 mg, fluoxetine 60 mg, fluvoxamine 300 mg, paroxetine 60 mg, and/or clomipramine 250 mg, since this disorder often requires higher doses than what would be seen if a major depression were being treated with the same medication. Each drug trial should be no less than 12 weeks. The Vietnam veteran's symptoms of autonomic hyperarousal are likely to respond to medications that inhibit adrenergic activity, such as beta-blockers. The bank teller presents with symptoms of generalized anxiety disorder (GAD). Tricyclics, SSRIs, and buspirone (a non-benzodiazepine antianxiolytic) are all effective with GAD, but because of the significant side effects of tricyclics, buspirone or SSRIs are most commonly used. In this case, buspirone would be the first treatment of choice, given that it has a very low incidence of side effects and a high rate of success with GAD. Benzodiazepines are also very effective with this disorder, but since they may be addictive, they are not recommended for people with a history of substance abuse. Alpha-adrenergic receptor antagonists (beta-blockers) are effective in the treatment of specific forms of social phobias such as fear of public speaking and fear of performing in front of an audience.

365. The answer is d. (*Kaplan and Sadock, pp 594-595.*) The combination of an SSRI (paroxetine) and a benzodiazepine (alprazolam) is considered optimal for this young woman with panic disorder. She is terrified of the panic attacks and needs swift relief. She has no history of substance abuse. Alprazolam will shut off the panic attacks almost immediately, and should be continued until the SSRI begins to take effect (typically several weeks). At that time, the patient can be slowly tapered off the alprazolam and continued on the SSRI.

Personality Disorders, Human Sexuality, and Miscellaneous Syndromes

Questions

366. A 7-year-old girl is brought to the physician because her parents note that she gets up at night and, still asleep, walks around the house for a few minutes before returning to bed. When she is forced to awaken during one of these episodes, she is confused and disoriented. Her parents are afraid that she will accidentally hurt herself during one of these episodes. Which of the following is the most appropriate intervention the physician should recommend?

a. Tell the parents to maintain a safe environment and monitor the patient's symptoms.
b. Start the patient on a low dose of benzodiazepines at night.
c. Start the patient on a low dose of a tricyclic antidepressant.
d. Tell the parents that the child would benefit from cognitive psychotherapy.
e. Admit the child to the hospital and obtain an EEG.

367. A 65-year-old woman lives alone in a dilapidated house, although her family members have tried in vain to move her to a better dwelling. She wears odd and out-of-fashion clothes and rummages in the garbage cans of her neighbors to look for redeemable cans and bottles. She is very suspicious of her neighbors. She was convinced that her neighbors were plotting against her life for a brief time after she was mugged and thrown onto the pavement by a teenager, but now thinks that this is not the case. She believes in the "power of crystals to protect me" and has them strewn haphazardly throughout her house. Which of the following is the most likely diagnosis?

a. Autism
b. Schizophrenia, paranoid type
c. Schizotypal personality disorder
d. Avoidant personality disorder
e. Schizoid personality disorder

368. A 17-year-old man comes to the physician because he has been falling asleep in inappropriate places, even though he has been getting enough rest at night. The patient states that he has fallen asleep while eating and driving. He notes that he stays asleep approximately 20 minutes and when he first wakes up, he is unable to move. He notes that sometimes he can even fall asleep while standing, and has been told by others that during those times he simply drops to the floor suddenly. He is fitted with a portable monitor, and it is found that during these episodes he enters an REM sleep stage immediately. Which of the following is the most likely diagnosis?

a. Narcolepsy
b. Sleep apnea
c. Primary hypersomnia
d. Kleine-Levin syndrome
e. REM sleep behavior disorder

369. A 32-year-old man is diagnosed with a major depression. He and his psychiatrist discuss starting an antidepressant. The patient is concerned about the chance for impairment of his ability to get an erection on these kinds of medications. Which of the following medications should the patient be started on to treat his depression but avoid these symptoms?

a. Imipramine
b. Phenelzine
c. Fluoxetine
d. Desipramine
e. Clomipramine

370. An attractive and well-dressed 22-year-old woman is arrested for prostitution, but on being booked at the jail, she is found to actually be a male. The patient tells the consulting physician that he is a female trapped in a male body and he has felt that way since he was a child. He has been taking female hormones and is attempting to find a surgeon who would remove his male genitals and create a vagina. Which of the following is the most likely diagnosis?

a. Homosexuality
b. Gender identity disorder
c. Transvestic fetishism
d. Delusional disorder
e. Schizophrenia

371. A 38-year-old man comes to his physician with complaints of impaired ejaculation. He is on the following medications: perphenazine, digoxin, and propranolol. He is also receiving methadone treatment and admits to periodic cannabis use. Which substance is the most likely culprit in his problems with ejaculation?

a. Perphenazine
b. Digoxin
c. Propanolol
d. Methadone
e. Cannabis

372. A 38-year-old married man comes to the psychiatrist because he felt his "sexuality is out of control." He notes that he never feels that he has had enough sex, even though he masturbates 3 to 4 times per day and has sex with his wife daily. He states he has tried to stop but feels he cannot control the behavior. He feels a lot of guilt about this, especially when he masturbates at his workplace. Which of the following medications would be most helpful to this man?

a. Benzodiazepines
b. SSRIs
c. Antipsychotics
d. Mood stabilizers
e. Buspirone

373. A demanding 25-year-old woman begins psychotherapy stating that she is both desperate and bored. She reports that for the past 5 or 6 years she has experienced periodic anxiety and depression and has made several suicidal gestures. She also reports a variety of impulsive and self-defeating behaviors and sexual promiscuity. She wonders if she might be a lesbian, though most of her sexual experiences have been with men. She has abruptly terminated two previous attempts at psychotherapy. In both cases she was enraged at the therapist because he was unwilling to prescribe anxiolytic medications. Which of the following is the most likely diagnosis?

a. Dysthymia
b. Histrionic personality disorder
c. Antisocial personality disorder
d. Borderline personality disorder
e. Impulse control disorder not otherwise specified

Questions 374 to 377

Match each patient's behavior with the most likely personality disorder. Each lettered option may be used once, more than once, or not at all.

a. Paranoid
b. Schizotypal
c. Schizoid
d. Narcissistic
e. Borderline
f. Histrionic
g. Antisocial
h. Obsessive-compulsive
i. Dependent
j. Avoidant

374. A 28-year-old woman begins seeing a psychiatrist because, she says, "I am just so very lonely." Her speech is excessively impressionistic and lacks specific detail. She flirts constantly with the physician and is "hurt" when the therapist does not notice her new clothes or hairstyle.

375. A 42-year-old man comes to the psychiatrist at the insistence of his boss because he constantly misses important deadlines. The man states that everyone at work is lazy and that no one lives up to his own standards for perfection. He is angry when the physician starts the interview 3 minutes later than the appointed time. He notes that he is always fighting with his wife because he is a "pack rat" and is unable to throw anything out. During the interview, he appears very rigid and stubborn.

376. A 34-year-old woman comes to the psychiatrist on the advice of her mother, because the patient still lives at home and will not make any decisions without her mother's reassurance. The patient's mother accompanies the patient to the appointment. She states that the patient becomes anxious when her mother must leave the home because the patient is terrified that her mother will die and the patient will have to take care of herself, something she feels incapable of doing.

377. A 25-year-old high school dropout has been arrested more than 12 times for various assault, fraud, and attempted murder charges. He has been in many physical fights, usually after he got caught cheating at cards. On examination, he seems relaxed and even cocky, and he shows no remorse for his actions.

Questions 378 to 380

Match each of the following descriptions of behavior with the temperament types that they characterize the most. Each lettered option may be used once, more than once, or not at all.

a. Harm avoidance
b. Novelty seeking
c. Reward dependence
d. Persistence

378. This temperament type is noted for being industrious and determined. Being lazy and spoiled is not a characteristic of this type.

379. This temperament type is noted for being open, sentimental, and affectionate. Opposite characteristics not seen in this temperament type are aloofness, detachment, and independence.

380. This temperament type is noted for being impulsive and extravagant. It is not noted for being deliberate or thrifty.

381. A 52-year-old man comes to the psychiatrist with complaints of problems sleeping. He has problems falling asleep, tossing and turning for several hours before finally getting to sleep. The next day the patient is tired, and this has caused him some problems at work. The patient denies signs or symptoms of major depression. Which of the following is the best sleep hygiene recommendation to help this patient sleep?

a. Eat a larger meal near bedtime.
b. Take daytime naps when possible.
c. Get up at the same time every day.
d. Watch television in bed until sleepy.
e. Begin a graded program of exercise in the early evening.

382. A 21-year-old man comes to the physician because of excessive sleepiness. He states that for the past 4 months he becomes so sleepy that he must sleep, even when he is in the middle of an important meeting. These episodes occur daily and the patient must sleep for 10 to 20 minutes at each episode. The patient also says that on several occasions he has had a sudden loss of muscle tone during which his knees become weak and he drops to the floor. He remains conscious during these episodes. He denies any substance abuse or medical problems. Which of the following is the most appropriate treatment to be started?

a. Benzphetamine
b. Valproic acid
c. Lithium
d. Modafinil
e. Nasal continuous positive airway pressure

383. A young librarian has been exceedingly shy and fearful of people since childhood. She longs to make friends, but even casual social interactions cause her a great deal of shame and anxiety. She has never been at a party, and she has requested to work in the least active section of her library, even though this means lower pay. She cannot look at her rare customers without blushing, and she is convinced that they see her as incompetent and clumsy. Which of the following personality disorders is most likely?

a. Schizotypal
b. Avoidant
c. Dependent
d. Schizoid
e. Paranoid

384. A 38-year-old man is seen by a psychiatrist because he has recurrent and intense sexually arousing fantasies involving wearing women's clothing. He notes that at first, he could wear women's underwear in his own home when he masturbated, and that this was sufficient. He now notes that he increasingly has the urge to wear women's clothes in public and masturbate somewhere less private. He comes in for help because he does not want to be caught at this behavior, though he is intensely attracted to it. He notes that he is a heterosexual, but that this cross-dressing behavior is sexually exciting to him. Which of the following disorders best describes this patient's symptoms?

a. Exhibitionism
b. Frotteurism
c. Sexual masochism
d. Transvestic fetishism
e. Gender identity disorder

385. A 48-year-old man has been unable to have intercourse with his wife of 20 years since she disclosed to him that she was having an affair with his younger and more attractive work partner. He continues having spontaneous nocturnal erections. This patient's sexual dysfunction is most likely caused by which of the following?

a. An organic disorder
b. A psychogenic determinant
c. A form of paraphilia
d. An irreversible psychodynamic process
e. A sexual identity disorder

386. A 21-year-old man comes to the psychiatrist with the complaint of chronic unhappiness. He states that his usual mood is unhappy, and his self-esteem is always low, and has been since childhood. He states he spends time brooding and worrying about all manner of issues, in particular over his own inadequacy. He states he is pessimistic about things as a general rule, and feels guilty a lot because he is "such a bad friend." He denies any unusual or stressful events occurring as a precipitant to this unhappiness. Which of the following is the most likely diagnosis?

a. Personality disorder NOS
b. Dysthymic disorder
c. Major depression
d. Avoidant personality disorder
e. Generalized anxiety disorder

387. A young woman presents to the emergency room vomiting bright red blood. Once she is medically stable, the intern who performs her physical examination notices that the enamel of her front teeth is badly eroded and her parotid glands are swollen. Which of the following best describes the source of these medical complications?

a. Inadequate caloric intake
b. Purging
c. Laxative abuse
d. Diuretic abuse
e. Ipecac toxicity

Questions 388 and 389

388. An off-Broadway actor consistently bores his friends and acquaintances by talking incessantly about his exceptional talent and his success on the stage. He does not seem to realize that other people do not share his high opinion of his acting talent and are not interested in his monologues. When a director criticizes the way he delivers his lines during rehearsal, the actor goes into a rage and accuses the director of trying to jeopardize his career out of jealousy. Which personality disorder represents the most likely diagnosis?

a. Histrionic
b. Narcissistic
c. Borderline
d. Paranoid
e. Antisocial

389. The patient in the vignette above seeks out a psychiatrist because, he says, "It is depressing when no one understands your talent." Which of the following treatments would be most appropriate?

a. Medication with an SSRI
b. Medication with a tricyclic antidepressant
c. Group psychotherapy with patients from a wide range of other diagnoses
d. Psychoanalysis
e. Psychodynamic psychotherapy

390. A 52-year-old woman is diagnosed with breast cancer that is metastatic to her bones. She comes to the psychiatrist for help in managing her depressed mood and anxiety secondary to this diagnosis. Which of the following would most likely indicate an increased vulnerability to suicide if found in this patient, in addition to her anxiety and depressed mood?

a. The extent of the cancer's spread to her bones
b. The location of the bone metastases to her bones
c. A feeling of a loss of control
d. How much pain she has with the metastases (even though it is currently well-controlled)
e. A history of social phobia

391. A 3-year-old girl's preferred make-believe game is playing house with her dolls. She loves to experiment with her mother's makeup and states that when she grows up, she will be a mommy. She is very offended when someone mistakes her for a boy. This scenario best demonstrates that which of the following is well established at this girl's age?

a. Theory of the mind
b. Sexual orientation
c. Gender identity
d. Gender neurosis
e. Gender dysphoria

Questions 392 to 395

Match each patient's symptoms with the correct diagnosis. Each lettered option may be used once, more than once, or not at all.

a. Primary hypersomnia
b. Narcolepsy
c. Sleep terror disorder
d. Circadian sleep disorder
e. Primary insomnia
f. Periodic limb movement disorder
g. Sleep apnea
h. Restless legs syndrome

392. A woman complains about her husband moving his legs constantly while he sleeps. She ends up being kicked several times every night. The husband has no memory of this nighttime activity, but he reports that he wakes up tired every morning despite getting what he considers an adequate amount of sleep (7 to 8 hours per night).

393. Because of her job's requirements, a per diem nurse works different shifts almost every week. She is constantly sleepy and fatigued. However, even when she has days off, she has great difficulty falling asleep at night and remaining asleep for more than 2 to 3 hours at a time.

394. For the past 2 years a 28-year-old man has found himself in many dangerous or embarrassing situations because of his inconvenient habit of falling abruptly asleep in the middle of any activity. Once he hit a pole because he fell asleep while driving. His wife still teases him for "taking a nap" while they were having sex. The man reports that he starts dreaming as soon as his eyes close, and when he wakes up, 10 to 20 minutes later, he feels wide awake and refreshed.

395. A young man has felt consistently sleepy during the day for as long as he can remember. Although he sleeps from 9 to 11 hours every night, he wakes up unrefreshed and needs to take a nap at least once a day in order to function. According to his wife and bed partner, he does not snore and he does not kick her while sleeping. Aside from the difficulties caused by his chronic sleepiness, his history is unremarkable.

Questions 396 to 399

Match each patient's behavior with the most likely personality disorder. Each lettered option may be used once, more than once, or not at all.
a. Paranoid
b. Schizotypal
c. Schizoid
d. Narcissistic
e. Borderline
f. Histrionic
g. Antisocial
h. Obsessive-compulsive
i. Dependent
j. Avoidant
k. No personality disorder apparent

396. A 24-year-old woman drops out of college after 2 weeks. When asked why, she states that although she would desperately like to have friends, she is afraid to approach anyone because "they would think I'm just a nerd." Furthermore, in the middle of a class, one of the professors asked her a question and she became extremely uncomfortable. She has never had a significant relationship with anyone other than her parents and sister.

397. A 32-year-old man comes to the psychiatrist because he is anxious about his new job. He notes that he previously held a job shelving books in the back of a library, but because of budget cuts he has been forced to interact with customers. He states he doesn't like being around people and prefers being by himself. He appears emotionally cold and detached during the interview.

398. A 19-year-old man comes to the psychiatrist because he can't leave the house without checking the stove, furnace, and water heater 25 times in a specific order. He notes that while he hates to perform this behavior, if he does not, he feels overwhelmingly anxious. It sometimes takes him 3 hours to leave the house in the morning because of this behavior.

399. A 32-year-old woman is admitted to the obstetrics ward to deliver a normal full-term infant. Ten hours after the delivery, she tries to steal the infant out of the nursery because she believes that the government of Myanmar is after her and will steal her child. When confronted by a nurse, she attempts to scratch the nurse and grab her child.

Personality Disorders, Human Sexuality, and Miscellaneous Syndromes

Answers

366. The answer is a. (*Moore and Jefferson, pp 234-235.*) Sleepwalking disorder is a parasomnia associated with slow-wave sleep. The patient is usually difficult to awaken, confused, and amnesic for the episode. Common in children, sleepwalking peaks between the ages of 4 and 8 years and usually disappears after adolescence. The person attempting to awaken the sleepwalker may be violently attacked. The severity of the disorder ranges from less than one episode per month without any problem to nightly episodes complicated by physical injury to the patient and others. There is no treatment recommended—rather, the goal is to continue to monitor the patient's symptoms and to maintain a safe environment until the disorder remits.

367. The answer is c. (*Jacobson and Jacobson, pp 61, 187.*) Schizotypal personality disorder, a cluster A disorder, is characterized by acute discomfort in close relationships, cognitive and perceptual distortions, and eccentric behavior beginning in early adulthood and present in a variety of contexts. Individuals with schizoid personality disorder do not present with the magical thinking, oddity, unusual perceptions, and odd appearance typical of schizotypal individuals. In schizophrenia, psychotic symptoms are much more prolonged and severe. Avoidant individuals avoid social interaction out of shyness and fear of rejection and not out of disinterest or suspiciousness. In autism, social interactions are more severely impaired and stereotyped behaviors are usually present.

368. The answer is a. (*Moore and Jefferson, pp 219-221.*) In narcolepsy, REM periods are not segregated in their usual rhythm during sleep but suddenly and repeatedly intrude into wakefulness. Nocturnal sleep shows a sleep-onset REM period or one that occurs very shortly after the onset of sleep. Among patients treated for this disorder, 15% to 30% also show some nocturnal myoclonus or sleep apnea. A majority of narcoleptics experience cataplexy (a sudden loss of muscle tone), hypnagogic hallucinations (dreamlike experiences occurring just before real sleep occurs), or sleep paralysis (brief paralysis occurring just before, or just after, the onset of sleep).

369. The answer is c. (*Kaplan and Sadock, p 696.*) All of the medications listed, except fluoxetine, have been shown to impair the achievement of erections. Fluoxetine, like the other SSRIs, may cause retarded ejaculation. This drug may also lower the sex drive or cause difficulty reaching orgasm in both sexes, probably secondary to the rise in serotonin levels that occur while taking it.

370. The answer is b. (*Moore and Jefferson, pp 191-205.*) In adolescents and young adults, gender identity disorder is characterized by strong cross-gender identification, a persistent discomfort with one's sex, and clinically significant distress or impairment. Such patients usually trace their conviction to early childhood, often live as the opposite sex, and seek sex reassignment surgery and endocrine treatment. These patients feel a sense of relief and appropriateness when they are wearing opposite-sex clothing. In contrast, patients with transvestic fetishism are sexually aroused by this behavior, and so typically only seek to wear clothing of the opposite sex during sexual situations. Homosexuality is not a diagnosis in *DSM-IV*. While some homosexuals cross-dress to seek a same-sex partner, they do not feel that they belong to the opposite sex, nor do they seek sex reassignment surgery.

371. The answer is a. (*Kaplan and Sadock, p 696.*) Perphenazine is known to cause impairment in ejaculation. The other drugs in the option list can cause impaired erections, but do not generally cause problems with ejaculation once an erection is achieved.

372. The answer is b. (*Kaplan and Sadock, pp 715-716.*) Because SSRIs can reduce the sex drive, these drugs can be used to treat sexual addiction. In this case, the drug's side effects can be used therapeutically. Medroxyprogesterone acetate also diminishes libido in men, so may also be effective in the treatment of sexually addictive behavior.

373. The answer is d. *(Ebert et al, pp 523-526.)* The patient's history and presenting symptoms are classic for the diagnosis of borderline personality disorder. Patients with borderline personalities present with a history of a pervasive instability of mood, relationships, and self-image beginning by early adulthood. Their behavior is often impulsive and self-damaging, their sexuality is chaotic, sexual orientation may be uncertain, and anger is intense and often acted out. Recurrent suicidal gestures are common. The shifts of mood usually last from a few hours to a few days. Patients often describe chronic feelings of boredom and emptiness.

374 to 377. The answers are 374-f, 375-h, 376-i, 377-g. *(Kaplan and Sadock, pp 791-812.)* Histrionic personality disorder is characterized by a chronic pattern of excessive emotionality and attention seeking. Patients with this disorder like to be the center of attention, and interaction with others is often inappropriately seductive. These patients may also use their physical appearance to draw attention to themselves. Speech is dramatic but superficial, and details are lacking. Patients are easily suggestible and influenced by others. Patients with obsessive-compulsive personality disorder are preoccupied with orderliness, perfection, and control. They are often so preoccupied with details, lists, and order that they lose sight of the forest for focusing on the trees. Their concern with perfectionism makes it difficult for them to complete projects in a timely manner. They are often perceived as rigid and stubborn. Patients with dependent personality disorder have a chronic and excessive need to be taken care of. This leads to submissive, clinging behavior in a desperate attempt to avoid being separated from the caretaker. These patients have difficulty making everyday decisions on their own and often need considerable reassurance before being able to do so. They are also unrealistically preoccupied with fears of being left alone to take care of themselves. Individuals with antisocial personality disorder display a chronic pattern of disregard for the rights of others, and they often violate them. They also are frequently irritable and aggressive, engaging in repeated physical assaults. They do not show remorse for their activities. This diagnosis is not made if the episodes of antisocial behavior occur exclusively during the course of schizophrenia or a manic episode.

378 to 380. The answers are 378-d, 379-c, 380-b. *(Kaplan and Sadock, pp 810-811.)* Four character traits have been described, each with their own characteristics and neurochemical and neurophysiologic substrates. Harm avoidance involves a heritable bias toward the inhibition of behavior in response to signals of punishment or nonreward. Those with high harm avoidance are generally uncertain, shy, with pessimistic worry in the face of problems. Persons high in novelty seeking are impulsive, curious, easily bored, and disorderly. Those high in reward dependence traits are tenderhearted, socially dependent, and sociable, while those low in this trait are practical, tough-minded, and indifferent if alone. Those with persistent temperament traits are hard-working and ambitious overachievers who view frustration and fatigue as a personal challenge.

381. The answer is c. *(Kaplan and Sadock, p 758.)* All of the options listed are the opposite of what one would recommend as a sleep hygiene measure, except for the recommendation to get up at the same time every day. Other sleep hygiene methods which can be recommended include: don't take central nervous system stimulants (coffee, nicotine, alcohol) before bedtime, avoid evening television—instead read or listen to the radio, try very hot 20-minute baths before bedtime, and practice evening relaxation routines such as progressive muscle relaxation.

382. The answer is d. *(Kaplan and Sadock, p 760.)* Modafinil (Provigil) has been approved by the FDA to reduce the number of sleep attacks and to lessen cataplexy (the sudden loss of muscle tone which is causing this patient's knees to buckle). Modafinil, like other stimulants, increases the release of monoamines, but also elevates hypothalamic histamine levels. Patients can develop tolerance to this drug and should be monitored closely while on it. It does lack some of the adverse side effects of psychostimulants, which were previously used to treat this disorder.

383. The answer is b. *(Jacobson and Jacobson, p 187.)* Avoidant personality disorder is characterized by pervasive and excessive hypersensitivity to negative evaluation, social inhibition, and feelings of inadequacy. Impairment can be severe because of social and occupational difficulties. Males and females are equally affected. The prevalence ranges from 0.5% to 1.5% in the general population. Among psychiatric outpatients, the prevalence is as high as 10%. Patients with avoidant personality disorder would like friends, but are so afraid that they will be rejected that they do not try to make them. Patients with schizoid personality disorders, by contrast, are socially isolated and prefer it that way.

384. The answer is d. (*Kaplan and Sadock, p 710.*) In transvestic fetishism, patients, usually heterosexual males, experience recurrent and intense sexual arousal while they are cross-dressing. Masturbation, with fantasies of sexual attractiveness while dressed as a woman, usually accompanies the cross-dressing. Wearing an article of women's clothing or dressing as a woman while having intercourse can also be sexually exciting for these patients. The condition often begins in childhood or early adolescence. Males with this disorder consider themselves to be male, but some have gender dysphoria. For diagnostic purposes, the behavior must persist over a period of at least 6 months.

385. The answer is b. (*Kaplan and Sadock, p 695.*) During periods of REM sleep, men experience penile erections defined as nocturnal penile tumescence (NPT). NPT studies can be helpful in differentiating patients with organic erectile problems from patients with psychogenic impotence. However, these findings are not absolute, since many men have both organic and psychological causes for their impotence and nocturnal erections may be decreased or absent in depression. Since this patient has NPT, it is likely that his impotence stems from a psychogenic determinant, which may be reversible with treatment.

386. The answer is a. (*Kaplan and Sadock, p 808.*) This patient does not meet the criteria for any one current personality disorder, and thus would receive a diagnosis of Personality Disorder NOS. Depressive personality disorder, part of *DSM-IV-TR's* research criteria, would actually fit this patient's symptomatology well. In this disorder, there is a pervasive pattern of depressive cognition and behavior which begins in early adulthood and persists throughout life. Patients with this personality disorder are pessimistic, anhedonic, self-doubting, and chronically unhappy. Their moods do not fluctuate as much as those with dysthymic disorder. Dysthymia is more episodic (though not as episodic as bipolar disorder or major depression) and usually occurs after some precipitating event. These patients may be at a great risk for developing dysthymia or a major depression.

387. The answer is b. (*Moore and Jefferson, pp 210-213.*) Chronic exposure of gastric juices through vomiting (purging) can cause severe erosion of the teeth and pathological pulp exposure in bulimic patients. Parotid gland enlargement is commonly observed in patients who binge and vomit. Esophageal tears, causing bloody emesis, can be a consequence of self-induced vomiting. The toxic effects of ipecac are cardiomyopathy and cardiac failure.

388 and 389. The answers are 388-b, 389-e. (*Kaplan and Sadock, p 803.*) The essential feature of narcissistic personality disorder is a pervasive pattern of grandiosity, need for admiration, and lack of empathy that begins by early adulthood. Individuals with this disorder overestimate their abilities, inflate their accomplishments, and expect others to share the unrealistic opinion they have of themselves. They believe they are special and unique and attribute special qualities to those with whom they associate. When they do not receive the admiration they think they deserve, people with narcissistic personality react with anger and devaluation. The prevalence of the disorder is estimated at less than 1% of the general population, and 50% to 75% of those diagnosed with narcissistic personality are males. In contrast with their outward appearance, individuals with this disorder have a very vulnerable sense of self. Criticism leaves them feeling degraded and hollow. Narcissistic traits are common in adolescence, but most individuals do not progress to develop narcissistic personality disorder. Treatment of narcissistic personality disorder is extremely difficult and requires a tactful therapist who can make confrontations, but do it gently. Forming an alliance with these patients can be very difficult. Medications do not work for this disorder. Psychoanalysis would be too intense for a patient with this disorder, and the abstinent stance would quickly drive the patient from therapy. Likewise, group therapy with a heterogeneous group would likely enrage a narcissist, who would be unable to take criticism from the other group members. Sometimes homogeneous groups of patients (a group with all narcissists, for example) might be able to work together therapeutically because it would help them understand their own maladaptive patterns as they watch others' behaviors.

390. The answer is c. (*Kaplan and Sadock, p 838.*) Suicide vulnerability factors in cancer patients include: depression and hopelessness, poorly controlled pain, feelings of loss of control, exhaustion, anxiety, family problems, and a positive family history of suicide.

391. The answer is c. (*Kaplan and Sadock, p 30.*) Gender identity refers to a person's perception of the self as male or female. Biological, social, and psychological factors contribute to its development. By 2½ years of age, children can consistently identify themselves as male or female and recognize others as male or female. Sexual orientation refers to the individual's sexual response to males, females, or both. Gender dysphoria refers to the discontent with their biological sex experienced by individuals with gender identity disorder. Theory of the mind refers to children's awareness that others have cognitive processes and an internal mental status similar to their own and to their ability to represent the mental status of others in their own mind.

392 to 395. The answers are 392-f, 393-d, 394-b, 395-a. *(Ebert et al, pp 470-495, 668-669.)* Periodic limb movement disorder, once called nocturnal myoclonus, is characterized by very frequent, stereotyped limb movements, most often involving the legs. The movements are accompanied by brief arousal and disruption of sleep pattern, although the individual suffering from the disorder is only aware of being chronically tired during the day. Interviewing bed partners helps clarify the diagnosis. It is differentiated from restless leg syndrome by the fact that in the latter, the patient is aware of much discomfort and a 'need to move' the legs. This discomfort can be alleviated by consciously moving the legs. Circadian sleep disorders are characterized by insomnia and chronic sleepiness. They are caused by a lack of synchrony between an individual's internal circadian sleep-wake cycles and the desired times of falling asleep and waking. The disorder can arise from an idiopathic variance in the periodic firing of the hypothalamic suprachiasmatic nucleus, which regulates the circadian cycles. The sleep cycles may be delayed, advanced, non-24-hour, or irregular. Traveling through several time zones and work shifts requiring considerable changes in sleep patterns is also responsible for the disorder. Narcolepsy is a disorder of unknown origin characterized by an irresistible urge to fall asleep. Sleep attacks last from 10 to 20 minutes and may take place at very inopportune times. Patients may also experience cataplexy (sudden loss of muscle tone triggered by a strong emotion), hypnagogic hallucinations (hallucinations associated with falling asleep), and sleep paralysis (the individual is unable to move on arousal, a benign but frightening experience that represents an intrusion of REM-sleep phenomena into wakefulness). Primary hypersomnia is a chronic or recurrent disorder characterized by daytime sleepiness, excessive nighttime sleep, and need for daytime naps. Polysomnographic studies show an increase in slow-wave sleep. To make this diagnosis, other causes of daytime sleepiness without sleep deprivation must be ruled out.

396 to 399. The answers are 396-j, 397-c, 398-k, 399-k. *(Ebert et al, pp 280, 513-516, 689.)* Avoidant personality disorder is characterized by an intense need for connection and social interaction with others, coupled with an intense fear of rejection. This fear causes patients to avoid any new or social situations that might be potentially embarrassing, and to feel extremely inadequate about the ability to start and maintain any kind of relationship. Conversely, patients with schizoid personality disorder, while every bit as isolated as those with avoidant personality disorder, like it that way. They rarely come to psychiatric attention because their social isolation is ego-syntonic. They do not like social relationships and usually prefer isolated activities. They have few, if any, friends. Question 398 refers to a patient with obsessive-compulsive disorder (not obsessive-compulsive personality disorder). Patients with OCD are characterized by obsessions (in this case, that there is something wrong with the stove, furnace, and water heater) and compulsions (the checking activity). These rituals can very much disturb a patient's life and are almost always ego-dystonic. Preventing the compulsions from occurring, however, causes a great deal of anxiety, as in this patient's case. Question 399 refers to a delusional patient (in this case, the patient has paranoid delusions). Delusions are fixed false beliefs that by their very definition cannot be changed. The magnitude of this patient's delusions is such that she acts on her paranoia by trying to steal her baby and scratch a nurse. Both obsessive-compulsive disorder and paranoid delusional disorder are often confused with obsessive-compulsive personality disorder and paranoid personality disorder, respectively.

Substance-Related Disorders

Questions

400. A 19-year-old man is brought to the emergency room by his distraught parents, who are worried about his vomiting and profuse diarrhea. On arrival, his pupils are dilated, his blood pressure is 175/105 mm Hg, and his muscles are twitching. His parents report that these symptoms started 2 hours earlier. For the past few days he has been homebound because of a sprained ankle, and during this time he has been increasingly anxious and restless. He has been yawning incessantly and has had a runny nose. From which of the following drugs is this man most likely to be withdrawing?

a. Heroin
b. Alcohol
c. PCP
d. Benzodiazepine
e. Cocaine

401. A 28-year-old woman is seen for postpartum blues by the psychiatrist. She states she is depressed because she "did this to her child." The infant has growth retardation, microphthalmia, short palpebral fissures, midface hypoplasia, a short philtrum, a thin upper lip, and microcephaly. Which is the most likely diagnosis of the mother (besides the postpartum blues)?

a. Bipolar disorder
b. Major depression
c. Hypochondriasis
d. Alcohol dependence
e. Cocaine dependence

Questions 402 and 403

402. A 50-year-old man is brought to the emergency department by ambulance. His respirations are shallow and infrequent, his pupils are constricted, and he is stuporous. He was noted to have suffered a grand mal seizure in the ambulance. On which of the following drugs is this man most likely to have overdosed?

a. Cocaine
b. LSD
c. An opiate
d. PCP
e. MDMA (Ecstasy)

403. After ensuring adequate ventilation for the patient in the previous vignette, which of the following interventions should be next?

a. Intravenous naloxone
b. Intravenous phenobarbitol
c. Intravenous diazepam
d. Forced diuresis
e. Intramuscular haloperidol

404. A 22-year-old man arrives at an emergency room accompanied by several friends. He is agitated, confused, and apparently responding to frightening visual and auditory hallucinations. The patient is put in restraints after he tries to attack the emergency room physician. The patient's friends report that he had "dropped some acid" 6 or 7 hours earlier. How much longer will intoxication with this substance last?

a. 1 to 6 hours
b. 8 to 12 hours
c. 14 to 18 hours
d. 20 to 24 hours
e. 26 to 30 hours

405. A college freshman, who has never consumed more than one occasional beer, is challenged to drink a large quantity of alcohol during his fraternity house's party. In a nontolerant person, signs of intoxication usually appear when the blood alcohol level reaches what range?

a. 20 to 30 mg/dL
b. 100 to 200 mg/dL
c. 300 mg/dL
d. 400 mg/dL
e. 500 mg/dL

406. A 27-year-old man is seen in the emergency room after getting into a fight at a local bar and being knocked unconscious. Upon his arrival in the emergency room, he is alert and oriented X 3. He states that he smokes marijuana 2 to 3 times per week and has done so for years. The last time he smoked was 2 days prior to admission to the emergency room. He also admits using PCP 5 days previously, and he took some of his wife's alprazolam the day prior to coming to the emergency room. Which of the following test results would likely be seen if the patient's urine were tested for substances of abuse in the emergency room?

	Marijuana	PCP	Alprazolam
a.	+	+	+
b.	+	−	+
c.	+	+	−
d.	−	−	−
e.	−	+	+

Questions 407 and 408

407. A 35-year-old man stumbles into the emergency room. His pulse is 100 beats/minute, his blood pressure is 170/95 mm Hg, and he is diaphoretic. He is tremulous and has difficulty relating a history. He does admit to insomnia the past two nights and sees spiders walking on the walls. He has been a drinker since age 19, but has not had a drink in 3 days. Which of the following is the most likely diagnosis?

a. Alcohol-induced psychotic disorder
b. Wernicke psychosis
c. Alcohol withdrawal delirium
d. Alcohol intoxication
e. Alcohol idiosyncratic intoxication

408. Which of the following is the most appropriate initial treatment for the patient from the previous vignette?

a. Intramuscular haloperidol
b. Intramuscular chlorpromazine
c. Oral lithium
d. Oral chlordiazepoxide
e. Intravenous naloxone

409. A 26-year-old woman presents to the psychiatrist with a 1-month history of severe anxiety. She states that 1 month ago she was a "normal, laid-back person." Since that time she rates her anxiety as an 8 on a scale of 1 to 10. She notes she is afraid to leave the house unless she checks that the door is locked at least 5 times. Which of the following would most likely cause these kinds of symptoms?

a. Alcohol intoxication
b. Amphetamine withdrawal
c. Caffeine withdrawal
d. Cocaine intoxication
e. Heroin intoxication

410. A 37-year-old woman is admitted to an inpatient treatment program for withdrawal from heroin. Eighteen hours after her last injection of heroin, she becomes hypertensive, irritable, and restless. She also has nausea, vomiting, and diarrhea. Which medication would be best to treat some of the symptoms of opioid withdrawal?

a. Chlordiazepoxide
b. Haloperidol
c. Paroxetine
d. Phenobarbital
e. Clonidine

411. Three policemen, with difficulty, drag an agitated and very combative young man into an emergency room. Once there, he is restrained because he reacts with rage and tries to hit anyone who approaches him. When it is finally safe to approach him, the resident on call notices that the patient has very prominent vertical nystagmus. Shortly thereafter, the patient has a generalized seizure. Which of the following substances of abuse is most likely to produce this presentation?

a. Amphetamine
b. PCP
c. Cocaine
d. Meperidine
e. LSD

Questions 412 and 413

412. A 64-year-old man is admitted to the emergency room after he was witnessed having a seizure on the sidewalk. Postictally, the patient was noted to be agitated and disoriented. Vital signs include: blood pressure 165/105 mm Hg, pulse 120 beats/minute. From the following list, which is the most likely diagnosis?

a. Cocaine intoxication
b. Alcohol withdrawal
c. PCP withdrawal
d. Cocaine withdrawal
e. Alcohol intoxication

413. In the vignette above, which of the following medications is most likely to be helpful to this patient postictally?

a. Librium IM
b. Haloperidol po
c. Clonidine po
d. Haloperidol IM
e. Lorazepam IM

414. A 20-year-old man is admitted to the emergency department after an automobile accident, in which his friend drove their car into a light pole. In the emergency department, the man smells strongly of alcohol, and his blood alcohol level is 300 mg/dL. However, he does not show any typical signs of intoxication. His gait is steady, his speech is clear, and he does not appear emotionally disinhibited. Which of the following is the most likely explanation for such a presentation?

a. The adrenaline generated in the patient because of the effects of the car crash has counteracted the alcohol in his system.
b. A value of 300 mg/dL is below the intoxication level.
c. The man has developed a tolerance to the effects of alcohol.
d. There has been a laboratory error.
e. The man has recently used cocaine, whose effects counteract the effects of alcohol intoxication.

415. A woman swallows two amphetamines at a party and quickly becomes disinhibited and euphoric. Afterward, she slaps a casual acquaintance because she takes a benign comment as a major offense and starts raving about being persecuted. What mechanism is most responsible for these behaviors?

a. Increased release of dopamine and norepinephrine in the synaptic cleft
b. Inhibition of catecholamine reuptake
c. Activation of NMDA receptors
d. Blockade of dopamine receptors
e. Sensitization of GABA receptors

416. A 25-year-old woman is dropped on the doorstep of a local emergency room by two men who immediately leave by car. She is agitated and anxious, and she keeps brushing her arms and legs "to get rid of the bugs." She clutches at her chest, moaning in pain. Her pupils are wide, and her blood pressure is elevated. Which of the following substances is she most likely using?

a. Alcohol
b. Heroin
c. Alprazolam
d. LSD
e. Cocaine

417. A 22-year-old woman comes to the physician with complaints of problems in sleeping. She notes that she has a hard time falling asleep, and when she does finally get to sleep, she awakens multiple times during the night. The patient says that this problem has been getting worse over the last 2 months. She states that she has also noted that she feels both nervous and fatigued during the day. Her mental status examination is otherwise normal. Toxicology screen is negative. Which of the following is the most likely diagnosis?

a. Sleep apnea
b. Marijuana intoxication
c. Caffeine-induced sleep disorder
d. ADHD
e. Major depression

418. A 22-year-old Asian woman becomes flushed and nauseated immediately after drinking half a glass of wine. She is noted to have slurred speech, ataxia, and nystagmus as well. She is brought to the emergency department by her concerned friends. Which of the following is the most likely diagnosis?

a. Conversion disorder
b. Panic disorder
c. Histrionic personality disorder
d. Factitious disorder with physical symptoms
e. Alcohol intoxication

419. A 35-year-old man comes to the psychiatrist for treatment of his heroin addiction. He has been an addict for over 6 years, and has been injecting heroin for 5 of those 6 years. Three previous attempts at quitting have all been unsuccessful. Which of the following medications is the best option for this man?

a. Methadone
b. Levomethadyl
c. Buprenorphine
d. Naloxone
e. Naltrexone

420. A 55-year-old man comes to his physician because he wants to stop smoking. He tells the physician that he is desperate to stop because his wife was just diagnosed with emphysema. The patient is willing to work with the physician on behavioral strategies to quit smoking but would also like some medications to help. Which of the following medications should the physician prescribe for this patient?

a. Lithium
b. Clonazepam
c. Methylphenidate
d. Bupropion
e. Amitriptyline

421. A 22-year-old man is brought to the emergency room after his friends noted he became agitated and was "acting crazy" at a party. The patient was belligerent and agitated in the emergency room as well. On physical examination, vertical nystagmus, ataxia, and dysarthria were noted. The patient has no previous mental or physical disorders. Which of the following is the best treatment option to give immediately?

a. Continuous nasogastric suction
b. Minimization of sensory inputs
c. Urinary acidification
d. Thorazine po
e. Naltrexone IM

422. A 16-year-old man with a long record of arrests for breaking and entering, assault and battery, and drug possession is found dead in his room with a plastic bag on his head. For several months he had been experiencing headaches, tremors, muscle weakness, unsteady gait, and tingling sensations in his hands and feet. These symptoms (and the manner in which the boy died) suggest that he was addicted to which of the following substances?

a. PCP
b. Cocaine
c. Methamphetamine
d. An inhalant
e. Heroin

423. A 13-year-old girl is brought to the emergency department by her mother because the girl thinks she is "going crazy." The girl states that at a friend's party several hours previously she was given a white tablet to take, which she did. She is now agitated and restless and convinced that she can fly. She also notes that she is having visual, auditory, and tactile hallucinations. On examination, she is noted to have tachycardia, tremors, hypertension, and mydriasis. Which of the following substances did she most likely ingest?

a. Cannabis
b. Heroin
c. Cocaine
d. MDMA (Ecstasy)
e. LSD

424. A 29-year-old man is brought to the psychiatrist by his wife because she is concerned about his increasing anger, irritability, and hostility over the past 4 months. The patient denies that any of these symptoms are problematic. On physical examination, the patient is noted to have bilateral muscle hypertrophy, especially in the upper body area, and an elevated fat-free mass index. Which of the following substances is most likely being abused by this man?

a. Amphetamines
b. Alcohol
c. Anabolic-androgenic steroids
d. Cocaine
e. PCP

425. A 16-year-old girl was brought to the emergency department by her mother, after the girl admitted that she had taken an unknown drug at a neighborhood party. The drug was identified as 3,4-methylenedioxymethamphetamine (MDMA), often known as Ecstasy. Which of the following side effects should the physician tell the patient's mother is common with use of this drug?

a. Anhedonia
b. Bruxism
c. Hypotension
d. An increased appetite
e. Suspiciousness and paranoia

Questions 426 to 428

Match each vignette with the correct term describing it. Each lettered option may be used once, more than once, or not at all.

a. Tolerance
b. Potentiation
c. Withdrawal
d. Dependence
e. Addiction
f. Substance abuse

426. A 22-year-old man continues to use alcohol on a once-weekly basis, despite the fact that every time he uses it he does something embarrassing, which he regrets. This has led him to lose some of his friends because they do not want to be around him when such behavior occurs.

427. A 36-year-old cocaine user notices that the longer he uses the drug, the more of it he requires to achieve the same effect.

428. A 22-year-old woman passes out in a bar after one drink of wine. She normally can drink two glasses before she feels any effects from the alcohol. Her psychiatrist has recently started her on a new medication for her nerves.

429. A 25-year-old man is brought to the emergency room after he became unconscious at a party. In the emergency room, the patient's respirations are 8 breaths/minute. and he is unresponsive. Eye witnesses at the party state the patient was observed taking several kinds of pills, drinking alcohol, and snorting cocaine. The patient is given a total of 1.5 mg of flumazenil, at which time he gradually awakens. Which of the following drugs was most likely the agent in this patient's unconsciousness?

a. An opioid
b. Cocaine
c. Alcohol
d. A benzodiazepine
e. A barbiturate

Substance-Related Disorders

Answers

400. The answer is a. (*Moore and Jefferson, p 80.*) Craving, anxiety, dysphoria, yawning, lacrimation, pupil dilatation, rhinorrhea, and restlessness are followed in more severe cases of withdrawal from short-acting drugs such as heroin or morphine by piloerection (cold turkey), twitching muscles and kicking movements of the lower extremities (kicking the habit), nausea, vomiting, diarrhea, low-grade fever, and increased blood pressure, pulse, and respiratory rate. Untreated, the syndrome resolves in 7 to 10 days. With longer-acting opiates, such as methadone, the onset of symptoms is delayed for 1 to 3 days after the last dose; peak symptoms do not occur until the third to eighth day, and symptoms may last for several weeks. Although very distressing, the opioid withdrawal syndrome is not life-threatening in healthy adults, but deaths have occurred in debilitated patients with other medical conditions.

401. The answer is d. (*Kaplan and Sadock, p 20.*) This woman is likely suffering from alcohol dependence because her child is showing the classic signs of a fetal alcohol syndrome. This syndrome affects approximately one-third of all infants born to women afflicted with alcoholism. Besides the signs this infant has, one can see delayed development, hyperactivity, attention deficits, learning disabilities, intellectual deficits, and seizures in these children.

402. The answer is c. (*Jacobson and Jacobson, pp 105-106.*) Severe opiate intoxication is associated with respiratory depression, stupor or coma, and sometimes pulmonary edema. Less severe intoxication is associated with slurred speech, drowsiness, and impaired memory or attention. Early on, the pupils are constricted, but they dilate if the patient becomes anoxic because of the respiratory depression. Blood pressure is typically reduced. Meperidine intoxication in a chronic user is often complicated by delirium or seizures caused by the accumulation of normeperidine, a toxic metabolite with cerebral irritant properties.

403. The answer is a. (*Kaplan and Sadock, pp 448-449.*) Naloxone, an opiate antagonist, is used to reverse the effects of opiates. The first treatment intervention, however, is to ensure that the patient is adequately ventilated. Tracheopharyngeal secretions should be aspirated, and the patient should be mechanically ventilated until naloxone is administered and a positive effect on respiratory rate is noticed. The usual initial dose of naloxone is 0.8 mg slowly administered intravenously. If there is no response, the dose can be repeated every few minutes. In most cases of opiate intoxication, 4 to 5 mg of naloxone (total dose) is sufficient to reverse the CNS depression. Buprenorphine may require higher doses. Diazepam is used to treat alcohol withdrawal symptoms. Forced diuresis is used in the treatment of salicylates and acetaminophen overdoses, not opiate intoxication. Haloperidol, an antipsychotic medication, is not used for the acute treatment of opiate intoxication.

404. The answer is a. (*Jacobson and Jacobson, pp 115-117.*) Most cases of intoxication with a hallucinogen are over within 8 to 12 hours, but prolonged drug-induced psychoses may occur, especially with phencyclidine (PCP), from which the psychosis may last several weeks.

405. The answer is a. (*Moore and Jefferson, pp 89-90.*) Behavioral changes, slowing of motor performance, and decrease in the ability to think clearly may appear with a blood alcohol level as low as 20 to 30 mg/dL. Most people show significant impairment of motor and mental performance when their alcohol levels reach 100 mg/dL. With blood alcohol concentration between 200 and 300 mg/dL, slurred speech is more intense and memory impairment, such as blackout and anterograde amnesia, becomes common. In a nontolerant person, a blood alcohol level over 400 mg/dL can produce respiratory failure, coma, and death. Because of tolerance, chronic heavy drinkers can present with fewer symptoms, even with blood alcohol levels greater than 500 mg/dL.

406. The answer is a. (*Kaplan and Sadock, p 261.*) The patient has admitted taking marijuana, PCP, and alprazolam (a benzodiazepine). These substances can be tested in the urine for, respectively, 3 days to 4 weeks (depending on use), 8 days, and 3 days. Thus, all three of these substances should show up as positive in this patient's urine.

407. The answer is c. (*Moore and Jefferson, pp 95-96.*) Alcohol withdrawal delirium (delirium tremens) is the most severe form of alcohol withdrawal.

In this syndrome, coarse tremor of the hands, insomnia, anxiety, agitation, and autonomic hyperactivity (increased blood pressure and pulse, diaphoresis) are accompanied by severe agitation, confusion, and tactile or visual hallucinations. When alcohol use has been heavy and prolonged, withdrawal phenomena start within 8 hours of cessation of drinking. Symptoms reach peak intensity between the second and third day of abstinence and are usually markedly diminished by the fifth day. In a milder form, withdrawal symptoms may persist for weeks as part of a protracted syndrome. Wernicke psychosis is an encephalopathy caused by severe thiamine deficiency, usually associated with prolonged and severe alcohol abuse. It is characterized by confusion, ataxia, and ophthalmoplegia. In alcohol hallucinosis, vivid auditory hallucinations start shortly after cessation or reduction of heavy alcohol use. Hallucinations may present with a clear sensorium and are accompanied by signs of autonomic instability less prominent than in alcohol withdrawal delirium.

408. The answer is d. (*Moore and Jefferson, pp 95-96.*) Benzodiazepines are the preferred treatment for alcohol withdrawal delirium, with diazepam and chlordiazepoxide (Librium) the most commonly used. Elderly patients or patients with severe liver damage may better tolerate intermediate-acting benzodiazepines such as lorazepam and oxazepam. Thiamine (100 mg) and folic acid (1 mg) are routinely administered to prevent CNS damage secondary to vitamin deficiency. Thiamine should always be administered prior to glucose infusion, because glucose metabolism may rapidly deplete patients' thiamine reserves in cases of long-lasting poor nutrition. When the patient has a history of alcohol withdrawal seizures, magnesium sulfate should be administered.

409. The answer is d. (*Kaplan and Sadock, pp 425-426.*) Cocaine-induced anxiety disorder can present with any of the symptoms occurring in this patient. Other symptoms of anxiety that can occur, and must be ruled out from the corresponding disorder, are panic disorder symptoms, or symptoms of phobias or obsessive-compulsive disorder.

410. The answer is e. (*Moore and Jefferson, p 80.*) Clonidine, an alpha-2-adrenergic receptor agonist, is used to suppress some of the symptoms of mild opioid withdrawal. Clonidine is given orally, starting with doses of 0.1 to 0.3 mg three or four times a day. In outpatient settings, a daily dosage above 1 mg is not recommended because of the risk of severe hypotension.

Clonidine is more effective on symptoms of autonomic instability, but is less effective than methadone in suppressing muscle aches, cravings, and insomnia. Clonidine is particularly useful in the detoxification of patients maintained on methadone.

411. The answer is b. (*Jacobson and Jacobson, pp 116-117.*) Phencyclidine (PCP) intoxication is characterized by neurological, behavioral, cardiovascular, and autonomic manifestations. Intoxicated patients are often agitated, enraged, aggressive, and scared. Because of their exaggerated and distorted sensory input, they may have unpredictable and extreme reactions to environmental stimuli. Nystagmus and signs of neuronal hyperexcitability (from increased deep tendon reflexes to status epilepticus) and hypertension are typical findings.

412 and 413. The answers are 412-b and 413-e. (*Kaplan and Sadock, p 399.*) Alcohol withdrawal delirium is a medical emergency, since untreated, as many as 20% of patients will die, usually as a result of a concurrent medical illness such as pneumonia, hepatic disease, or heart failure. Symptoms of this delirium include: autonomic hyperactivity, hallucinations, and fluctuating activity levels, ranging from acute agitation to lethargy. The best treatment for this delirium is, of course, prevention. However, once it appears, chlordiazepoxide should be given orally, or if this is not possible (as in this case), lorazepam should be given IV or IM. Antipsychotic medications should be avoided, since they may further lower the seizure threshold.

414. The answer is c. (*Moore and Jefferson, pp 80, 86.*) After prolonged use, most drugs of abuse (and some medications) produce adaptive changes in the brain that are manifested by a markedly diminished responsiveness to the effects of the substance that has been administered over time, a phenomenon called tolerance. *Anyone* who does not show signs of intoxication with an alcohol level of 150 mg/dL has developed a considerable tolerance.

415. The answer is a. (*Kaplan and Sadock, pp 407-412.*) The main mechanism of action of amphetamines is the release of stored monoamines in the synaptic cleft. Cocaine inhibits the reuptake of the neurotransmitters released in the synapse. Benzodiazepines and barbiturates act by increasing the affinity of GABA type A receptors for their endogenous neurotransmitter, GABA. NMDA aspartate receptors are activated by PCP. Antipsychotic medications act by blocking dopamine receptors.

416. The answer is e. (*Kaplan and Sadock, pp 421-428.*) Cocaine intoxication is characterized by euphoria but suspiciousness. Agitation, anxiety, and hyperactivity are also typical presenting symptoms. Signs of sympathetic stimulation, such as tachycardia, cardiac arrhythmias, hypertension, pupillary dilatations, perspiration, and chills are also present. Visual and tactile hallucinations, including hallucinations of bugs crawling on the skin, are present in cocaine-induced delirium. Among the most serious acute medical complications associated with the use of high doses of cocaine are coronary spasms, myocardial infarcts, intracranial hemorrhages, ischemic cerebral infarcts, and seizures.

417. The answer is c. (*Kaplan and Sadock, p 415.*) Caffeine is a stimulant that can cause a sleep disorder when it is used in excess. Patients may not recognize caffeine as a "drug" so may answer negatively to questions about drug use. Therefore, a question about caffeine use should be asked specifically to all patients presenting with difficulty sleeping. The sleep disorder caused by caffeine can produce a delay in falling asleep, an inability to remain asleep, and/or early morning awakening.

418. The answer is e. (*Kaplan and Sadock, p 396.*) Among Asian men and women, 10% lack the form of acetaldehyde dehydrogenase responsible for metabolizing low blood concentrations of acetaldehyde (they are homozygous for an inactive form of the enzyme). Approximately 40% of Asian men and women are heterozygous for this specific enzyme variation. Because of the rapid accumulation of acetaldehyde, homozygous individuals develop facial flushing, nausea, and vomiting after ingestion of small quantities of alcohol, which are the common side effects of alcohol intoxication and occur much earlier than the norm. Heterozygous individuals can tolerate some alcohol but are more sensitive to its effects. This enzyme variation is found only in people of Asian descent.

419. The answer is a. (*Kaplan and Sadock, p 449.*) This patient is likely to do better with methadone as he attempts to get rid of his heroin addiction. Methadone has the advantage that it frees addicts from needing to inject opioid substances, reducing the chance of HIV infection. It produces less drowsiness and less euphoria, so addicts can be functional and thus become employed, rather than spending their lives searching for enough cash for their next injection. The patient will still be dependent on a narcotic, but it is a more likely successful treatment regimen than quitting narcotics completely after three previously unsuccessful attempts.

420. The answer is d. (*Kaplan and Sadock, pp 441-442.*) A variety of psychopharmacologic agents, including clonidine, antidepressants, and buspirone, have been used with some success in the treatment of nicotine dependence. Bupropion (Zyban) was approved by the FDA in 1996 for this use. Nicotine replacement patches and gum can also be used and then tapered off slowly to reduce the symptoms of nicotine withdrawal. A new drug, varenicline (Chantix) has also been released to the market. It is a non-nicotine prescription medicine specifically developed to help adults quit smoking. Chantix contains no nicotine, but targets the same receptors that nicotine does. Chantix is believed to block nicotine from these receptors.

421. The answer is b. (*Kaplan and Sadock, pp 451-453.*) PCP disrupts sensory input, so those intoxicated with it can be extremely unpredictable with regard to any environmental stimuli. Thus, the best immediate treatment option for this patient is the minimization of such stimuli. Continuous NG suction can be overly intrusive and cause electrolyte imbalances. Urinary acidification can increase the risk of renal failure secondary to rhabdomyolysis, and so is both ineffective and potentially dangerous.

422. The answer is d. (*Kaplan and Sadock, pp 435-438.*) Inhalant abuse is associated with very serious medical problems. Hearing loss, peripheral neuritis, paresthesias, cerebellar signs, and motor impairment are common neurological manifestations. Muscle weakness caused by rhabdomyolysis, irreversible hepatic and renal damage, cardiovascular symptoms, and gastrointestinal symptoms such as vomiting and hematemesis are also common with chronic severe abuse.

423. The answer is e. (*Kaplan and Sadock, pp 428-434.*) Patients ingesting LSD may have a wide variety of sensory disturbances, and because of the sympathomimetic effects of the drug, may experience tremors, hypertension, tachycardia, mydriasis, hyperthermia, sweating, and blurry vision. Patients may die when they act on their false perceptions (in this case, the belief that the patient can fly) or accidentally kill themselves. When the subject is not clear about which drug was taken, the unexpected sensory disturbances can be quite terrifying, and patients can fear losing their minds, as in this case.

424. The answer is c. (*Kaplan and Sadock, pp 462-463.*) Steroids may cause a variety of mood effects, including euphoria and hyperactivity. However, they can also cause irritability, increased anger, hostility, anxiety, and depression.

There is also a correlation between steroid use and violence. These substances are addictive, and when addicts stop taking steroids, they may become depressed, anxious, and concerned about their bodies' appearance.

425. The answer is b. *(Kaplan and Sadock, pp 411-412.)* MDMA (Ecstasy) was tried in the 1970s as an adjunct to psychotherapy and later became popular as a recreational drug. After ingestion, there is an initial phase of disorientation, followed by a "rush" that includes increased blood pressure and pulse rate as well as sweating. Users experience euphoria, increased self-confidence, and peaceful feelings of empathy and closeness to other people; effects usually last 4 to 6 hours. MDMA decreases appetite. It has been associated with bruxism (grinding of the teeth), shortness of breath, cardiac arrhythmia, and death.

426 to 428. The answers are 426-f, 427-a, 428-b. *(Kaplan and Sadock, pp 381-385.)* These terms are commonly confused or used ambiguously. Substance abuse describes a maladaptive behavioral pattern characterized by recurrent use in spite of academic, social, or work problems; use in situations in which changes in mental status may be dangerous (driving); and recurrent substance-related legal problems. Tolerance refers to the pharmacological adaptation because of which a larger dose of a drug becomes necessary over time to achieve the same effect. Withdrawal refers to a substance-specific syndrome that occurs after the cessation of the substance whose use has been heavy and prolonged. An example of the use of potentiation for clinical benefit is the coadministration of a benzodiazepine and an antipsychotic to an agitated psychotic patient. Both medications can be administered at lower doses when used together than either could if used alone. Dependence is a condition in which withdrawal symptoms occur if the drug is stopped, usually leading to further drug use despite adverse consequences. With respect to drugs of abuse, tolerance and dependence often coexist.

429. The answer is d. *(Kaplan and Sadock, p 1020.)* Flumazenil is used to counteract the effects of benzodiazepine receptor agonists. It is administered via IV and has a half-life of approximately 10 to 15 minutes. Common adverse side effects of its use include: nausea, vomiting, dizziness, agitation, emotional lability, fatigue, impaired vision, and headache. The most serious adverse effect is the precipitation of seizures, most likely to occur when given to a person with a preexisting seizure disorder.

Psychopharmacology and Other Somatic Therapies

Questions

Questions 430 and 431

430. A 40-year-old man comes to the emergency room with symptoms of tachycardia, diaphoresis, mydriasis, and hyperthermia. He also shows muscle twitching and clonus. His medications include a protease inhibitor (for AIDS) and fluoxetine 20 mg daily which was started 1 week ago. What is the problem that most likely brought this man into the emergency room?

a. AIDS dementia
b. Encephalopathy
c. Serotonin syndrome
d. Delirium
e. Anticholinergic crisis

431. In the vignette above, what is the most likely pathophysiology of this disease process?

a. The pathophysiology is unknown.
b. The patient overdosed on fluoxetine.
c. The patient overdosed on his protease inhibitor.
d. There is increased sensitivity to these medicines with decreased organic capacity, leading to a delirium.
e. The protease inhibitor inhibits the metabolism by P450, thus increasing the level of the SSRI.

432. A 32-year-old man is started on Lithium after being diagnosed with bipolar disorder. His psychiatrist explains the risks and benefits of the drug and tells the patient that the drug can affect several organs in the body and he will need blood tests every 6 months. Which of the following labs should be drawn that often on this patient?

a. T₃RU.
b. TSH.
c. BUN.
d. CBC.
e. No labs need to be drawn with this frequency.

433. An 85-year-old man is brought to the psychiatrist by his wife. She states that for the last 4 months, since the death of his son, the patient has been unable to sleep, has lost 20 lb, has crying spells, and in the last week has been starting to talk about suicide. She notes that he has numerous other medical problems, including prostatic hypertrophy, hypertension, insulin-dependent diabetes, and a history of myocardial infarction. Which of the following medications is most appropriate for the treatment of this patient?

a. Doxepin
b. Clonazepam
c. Sertraline
d. Tranylcypromine
e. Amitriptyline

434. A 12-year-old boy is very distraught because every time he thinks or hears the word God or passes in front of a church, swear words pop into his mind against his will. He also feels compelled to repeat the end of every sentence twice and to count to 20 before answering any question. If he is interrupted, he has to start from the beginning. Which of the following medications has been proven effective with this disorder?

a. Alprazolam
b. Clomipramine
c. Propranolol
d. Phenobarbital
e. Lithium

435. A 7-year-old boy is brought to the physician with a 1-year history of making careless mistakes and not listening in class and at home. He is easily distracted and forgetful and loses his schoolbooks often. He is noted to be fidgety, talking excessively, and interrupting others. Which of the following medications is most likely to help with this boy's symptoms?

a. Haloperidol
b. Alprazolam
c. Lithium
d. Methylphenidate
e. Paroxetine

436. A patient with schizophrenia is being treated with clozapine. He is told he needs an initial CBC, then weekly CBCs for the first 6 months of treatment, which he agrees to do. Four months into the therapy, the patient's WBC count is noted to be 3250 per mm^3. The patient complains of a mild sore throat. Which of the following actions should the physician take first?

a. Start twice per week CBCs with differential counts. Continue the clozapine.
b. Interrupt the clozapine therapy. Get daily CBCs with differential. Restart the clozapine after the CBC normalizes.
c. Discontinue the clozapine immediately. Place the patient in protective isolation.
d. Consult with a hematologist to determine the appropriate antibiotic therapy.
e. Repeat the CBC in 1 week, if the level of WBCs drops again, discontinue clozapine.

437. A 36-year-old man is admitted to the hospital after a suicide attempt, in which he swallowed his entire bottle of lithium pills. In the emergency room, he is noted to be stuporous, with a lithium level of 4.5 meq/L. His urine output is noted to be less than one-half what would normally be expected for a patient of his age. Which of the following procedures should be performed next?

a. Administration of normal saline IV
b. Emergency dialysis
c. Administration of benztropine IM
d. Cardiac monitoring
e. Administration of flumazenil

Questions 438 and 439

438. A 32-year-old man comes to the physician with complaints of insomnia. He states for the past 3 weeks he has had difficulty going to sleep, though once he finally gets to sleep, he stays asleep without difficulty. The patient states that he is having no other difficulties. The patient has a past history of alcohol dependence, though he has been sober for over 3 years. Which of the following medications is the best choice to prescribe to help the patient with his sleep?

a. Ramelteon
b. Trazodone
c. Zolpidem
d. Triazolam
e. Zaleplon

439. In the patient in the vignette above, it is most important to rule out which of the following medical problems before using the desired sleep aid?

a. Mild COPD
b. Kidney failure
c. Severe hepatic impairment
d. Heart disease
e. Seizure disorder

440. A 57-year-old woman is seeing a psychiatrist for her bipolar disorder. She is started on carbamazepine. Which of the following tests should be done every 3 months during her second year of treatment with this drug?

a. Platelet count
b. Serum electrolytes
c. SGOT
d. ECG
e. Urinalysis

441. A 52-year-old woman is brought to the emergency room after her husband finds her unresponsive at home. The patient left behind a suicide note, and two empty bottles of pills (sertraline and lorazepam) plus an empty bottle of vodka were found next to the patient. In the emergency room the patient's vital signs are: blood pressure 90/60 mm Hg, pulse 60 beats/minute, respirations 6 breaths/minute. Which of the following medications is most likely to be helpful in the emergency room setting in this situation?

a. Acamprosate
b. Zolpidem
c. Flumazenil
d. LAAM
e. Disulfiram

442. A 32-year-old woman comes to the psychiatrist because she is "tired of worrying all the time." She notes that she can't control the worrying, and that she worries about everything; money, her children, who will run the country, "even stupid things." She also reports she has difficulty sleeping and concentrating, and is frequently irritable. She reports that her physician put her on a benzodiazepine to help her sleep, but that it "doesn't work." She requests buspirone, which she read about on-line. Why is this drug a poor choice for this patient?

a. Her disorder is better treated by another drug.
b. She has been taking benzodiazepines.
c. No drug has been proven effective for her disorder.
d. The first-line treatment for this disorder is an SSRI.
e. She needs psychotherapy before any drug can be helpful.

Questions 443 and 444

443. A 48-year-old woman with a past history of recurrent psychotic depression is admitted to a locked ward during a relapse. On the day of admission, she is placed on nortriptyline 50 mg and risperidone 2 mg at bedtime. Ten days later, the patient reports with great concern that her nipples are leaking. Which class of medications is most commonly known to cause this condition?

a. Benzodiazepines
b. Neuroleptics
c. Serotonin reuptake inhibitors
d. Antiseizure medications with mood-stabilizing properties
e. Beta-blockers

444. Which of the following mechanisms is responsible for the condition in the previous vignette?

a. Excessive release of monoamines in the synaptic cleft
b. Blockage of serotonin reuptake
c. Activation of NMDA receptors
d. Dopamine receptor blockade
e. Sensitization of GABA receptors to the agonistic effects of endogenous GABA

445. A 44-year-old woman comes to the psychiatrist for treatment of a major depression. Her BMI is 28. She states she has lost 50 lb in the past year and is determined not to gain it back. Which of the following medications would be the best choice to treat her depression, given these circumstances?

a. Amitriptyline
b. Doxepin
c. Nortriptyline
d. Phenelzine
e. Sertraline

446. A 41-year-old woman comes to the physician for her yearly physical examination. She states her medications include hydrochlorothiazide, omeprazole, and atorvastatin (Lipitor). In addition, she is taking St. John's wort and ginseng. These two alternative medications are most commonly used by many patients for which of the following symptoms?

a. As an antispasmodic
b. For depressed mood
c. To improve appetite
d. To improve concentration
e. For headaches

447. A 30-year-old woman is diagnosed as bipolar. At the same time that this illness is diagnosed, it is discovered that she is pregnant. Which of the following drugs has the highest risk to the fetus?

a. Valproic acid
b. Lithium
c. Chlorpromazine
d. Haloperidol
e. Fluoxetine

448. A 25-year-old woman with bipolar disorder develops a high fever with chills, bleeding gums, extreme fatigue, and pallor 3 weeks after starting on carbamazepine. Which of the following is she most likely experiencing?

a. Stevens-Johnson syndrome
b. Acute aplastic anemia
c. Serotonin syndrome
d. Neuroleptic malignant syndrome
e. Malignant hyperthermia

449. A 28-year-old woman is brought to the emergency room after her mother called an ambulance. The patient has a history of chronic schizophrenia, which is being treated with antipsychotics. The dosage was recently increased on these medications. In the emergency room the patient has a temperature of 39.44°C (103°F), is rigid, and has a blood pressure alternating between 120/65 and 100/45 mm Hg. Which of the following levels should be closely monitored?

a. WBC
b. Creatine phosphokinase (CPK)
c. Platelet levels
d. Creatinine clearance
e. Antipsychotic levels

450. A 24-year-old woman comes to the emergency room with complaints of feeling "stiffness and twisting" of her neck and jaw. She describes these symptoms as very uncomfortable and completely involuntary. She has not had these symptoms previously. Her medications include: lithium and trifluophenazine. The patient looks uncomfortable, and her jaw and neck are tense and twisted. In an emergency room setting, which of the following actions should the physician take first?

a. Gastric lavage for lithium overdose
b. Benztropine IM
c. Diphenhydramine po
d. Trifluophenazine po
e. Draw a lithium level

451. A 42-year-old man is diagnosed with a psychotic depression and is started on imipramine and perphenazine. When he develops a dystonia, he is begun on benztropine 2 mg/day. One week later, his wife reports that the patient has become unusually forgetful and seems disoriented at night. On physical examination, the man appears slightly flushed, his skin and palms are dry, and he is tachycardic. He is oriented to name and place only. He showed none of these symptoms during his last appointment. Which of the following is the most likely diagnosis?

a. Anticholinergic syndrome
b. Neuroleptic malignant syndrome
c. Extrapyramidal side effect
d. Akathisia
e. Dementia

452. A 56-year-old woman who was diagnosed with paranoid schizophrenia in her early twenties has received daily doses of various typical neuroleptics for many years. For the past 2 years, she has had symptoms of tardive dyskinesia. Discontinuation of the neuroleptic is not possible because she becomes aggressive and violent in response to command hallucinations when she is not medicated. Which of the following actions should be taken next?

a. Start the patient on benztropine.
b. Start the patient on amantadine.
c. Start the patient on propranolol.
d. Start the patient on diphenhydramine.
e. Switch the patient to clozapine.

453. A 27-year-old man is started on several new medications for treatment of a depressed mood. He returns to the physician's office after 2 weeks stating that on two separate occasions his wife noted that he got up from bed, went to the kitchen, and consumed large quantities of food in the middle of the night. The patient has no memory of this behavior. Which one of the following drugs could have been given that can produce this paradoxical response?

a. Sertraline
b. Lorazepam
c. Zolpidem
d. Fluoxetine
e. Valproic acid

454. A 23-year-old man was admitted to a psychiatric inpatient service for treatment of auditory hallucinations of a command nature, telling him to kill himself. He is started on perphenazine. One day later he is noted to be increasingly anxious and pacing the halls. He states he feels as if he "has to move" and that pacing helps a little. He denies that his mind is racing. Which of the following actions should the psychiatrist take next?

a. Increase the patient's perphenazine.
b. Discontinue the perphenazine.
c. Give Vitamin E po.
d. Give diphenhydramine.
e. Give propranolol.

Questions 455 and 456

455. A 53-year-old man is admitted to psychiatry after a serious suicide attempt. He remains nearly catatonic on the unit, refusing to either eat or drink. He also remains quite suicidal, and requires one-to-one observation at all times. Which of the following is the most appropriate treatment?

a. Tricyclic + SSRI in combination
b. SSRI at a higher than normal dose
c. SSRI + antipsychotic
d. Transcranial magnetic stimulation
e. ECT

456. The patient in the vignette above is to be given ECT. Which of the following anesthetic agents should be used prior to the procedure?

a. Fentanyl
b. Chloral hydrate
c. Methohexital
d. Alprazolam
e. Amobarbital

457. A 72-year-old man develops acute urinary retention and blurred vision after taking an antidepressant for 3 days. Which of the following medications is most likely to cause such side effects?

a. Venlafaxine
b. Paroxetine
c. Bupropion
d. Nefazodone
e. Amitriptyline

458. A 43-year-old woman comes to the physician because she wants a medication to help her stop smoking. On history, it is also found that she meets the criteria for a hypoactive sexual desire disorder. Which of the following medications will be the most helpful for this patient?

a. SSRI + nicotine patch
b. Bupropion
c. SSRI alone
d. Carbamazepine
e. MAOI + nicotine patch

459. A 9-year-old girl is brought to the physician because she is noted to be easily distractible and fidgety and is generally difficult to get focused at school. The physician starts the girl on Ritalin. Which of the following cautions about the drug should the physician give the child's mother?

a. Do not give the medication with food.
b. Do not give the medication after noon.
c. Do not give the medication with other medications.
d. The medication may cause photosensitivity.
e. The medication may precipitate mania.

Questions 460 and 461

460. A 34-year-old woman with a history of alcohol abuse has her first relapse after 2 years of sobriety. Fearing that she may not be able to stay away from alcohol, she asks her primary care physician to prescribe disulfiram. The following week, she arrives at the emergency room with facial flushing, hypotension, tachycardia, nausea, and vomiting. She denies any recent ingestion of alcohol. Which of the following is most likely to have caused her symptoms?

a. Aged cheese
b. Cough syrup
c. An overripe mango
d. Two 30-mg tablets of pseudoephedrine
e. A bar of chocolate

461. The effect of disulfiram depends on which of the following mechanisms?

a. Monoamine oxidase inhibition
b. Lactate dehydrogenase inhibition
c. Dopamine receptor blockade
d. α2-Receptor antagonism
e. Acetaldehyde dehydrogenase inhibition

462. A 24-year-old man comes to see his physician after he is involved in a serious car crash because he fell asleep while driving. For several years, he has had severe daytime sleepiness, episodes of falling asleep without warning, and hypnagogic hallucinations. Which of the following is the most appropriate medication for this patient?

a. Melatonin
b. Clonazepam
c. Methylphenidate
d. Thyroxine
e. Bromocriptine

463. For several weeks, a 72-year-old retired physician with Parkinson disease and mild dementia has been talking about "those horrible people that come to bother me every night." He is convinced that someone is plotting against him, and he has nailed his window shut for fear of intruders. More recently, he has started showing signs of thought disorder, mostly in the evening and at night. Which of the following antipsychotic medications is best to use on a patient with Parkinson disease?

a. Haloperidol
b. Perphenazine
c. Fluphenazine
d. Clozapine
e. Chlorpromazine

464. A 38-year-old woman is being seen by her psychiatrist for the treatment of her bipolar disorder. She is taking carbamazepine and sertraline and has been well controlled. At her last visit, her carbamazepine level was above therapeutic. She states she has not taken extra, but has recently started taking another medication prescribed by her physician. Which of the following medications is most likely to increase carbamazepine concentrations in this manner?

a. Theophylline
b. Erythromycin
c. Warfarin
d. Cisplatin
e. Hormonal contraceptives

465. A 29-year-old woman with a previous diagnosis of bipolar disorder is hospitalized during an acute manic episode. She is elated, sexually provocative, and speaks very fast, jumping from one subject to another. She tells the nurses that she has been chosen by God to be "the second virgin Mary." BUN, creatinine, electrolytes, TSH, and an ECG are within normal limits. Treatment with lithium is begun. Within what time interval does this medication come to steady state with regular administration?

a. Less than 24 hours
b. 1 to 4 days
c. 5 to 8 days
d. 2 to 3 weeks
e. 1 to 2 months

466. A 25-year-old woman with schizophrenia is started on an antipsychotic medication to control her symptoms. While her hallucinations decrease on the medication, she notes that she feels as if her "skin is crawling" and her legs "want to move by themselves." She is very uncomfortable with these symptoms and paces the floor continuously because of them. Her psychiatrist recommends propranolol to help control these symptoms. For which of the following comorbid medical conditions would this medication be contraindicated in this patient?

a. Obesity
b. Asthma
c. Alcohol abuse
d. Hypertension
e. Breast cancer

467. Which of the following hormones is most commonly used in the adjuvant treatment of depression?

a. Progesterone
b. Cortisol
c. ACTH
d. Levothyroxine
e. Prolactin

468. A patient with refractory schizophrenia has been almost free of active psychotic symptoms and has been functioning considerably better since he was placed on clozapine 500 mg/day, but he has experienced two episodes of grand mal seizure. Which of the following steps should be taken next?

a. Discontinue the clozapine and begin another antipsychotic.
b. Decrease the clozapine.
c. Stop the clozapine and start valproic acid.
d. Add Tegretol to the clozapine.
e. Temporarily stop the clozapine and start phenobarbital.

469. A patient reports that she has become depressed with the onset of winter every year for the past 6 years. Which of the following treatments is most likely to be helpful?

a. Phototherapy
b. Biofeedback
c. Electroconvulsive therapy
d. Benzodiazepines
e. Steroid medication

470. A 19-year-old girl is taken hostage with other bystanders during an armed robbery. She is freed by police intervention after 10 hours of captivity, but only after she has witnessed the shooting death of two of her captors. Months after this event, she has flashbacks and frightening nightmares. She startles at every noise and experiences acute anxiety whenever she is reminded of the robbery. Which of the following medications would most likely help decrease this patient's hyperarousal?

a. Clonidine
b. Methylphenidate
c. Bupropion
d. Valproate
e. Thioridazine

471. A 72-year-old man with a long history of recurrent psychotic depression is hospitalized during a relapse. He has prostatic hypertrophy, coronary heart disease, and recurrent orthostatic hypotension. Which of the following is the most appropriate antipsychotic medication for this patient?

a. Chlorpromazine
b. Clozapine
c. Thioridazine
d. Haloperidol
e. Olanzapine

472. A 47-year-old businessman who has taken paroxetine 40 mg/day for 6 months for depression leaves for a 2-week business trip overseas and forgets his medication at home. Since his depression has been in full remission for at least 3 months, he decides to stop the treatment without talking with his psychiatrist. Two days later, he becomes very irritable, tearful, dizzy, and nauseated. He shivers and feels like he has a bad cold. Which of the following is the most likely cause of such symptoms?

a. Relapse of his major depression
b. Serotonin syndrome
c. SSRI discontinuation syndrome
d. Manic episode
e. Jet lag

473. The benzodiazepines' action depends on their interaction with which of the following receptors?

a. GABA
b. Serotonin
c. NMDA-glutamate
d. Dopamine
e. Acetylcholine

Questions 474 and 475

474. A 42-year-old woman with atypical depression who has responded well to an MAOI presents to an emergency room with severe headache. Her blood pressure is 180/110 mm Hg. She states that she has been carefully avoiding high-tyramine foods as she was told, but she admits that a friend gave her two tablets of a cold medication shortly before her symptoms started. Which of the following over-the-counter medications is contraindicated with MAOI treatment?

a. Pseudoephedrine
b. Acetaminophen
c. Diphenhydramine
d. Ibuprofen
e. Guaifenesin

475. If the woman's symptoms from the vignette above were caused by a dietary indiscretion, which of the following foods would be the most probable cause?

a. A slice of pepperoni pizza
b. A bagel with cream cheese
c. A chocolate candy bar
d. A glass of white wine
e. A cup of coffee

476. A 28-year-old woman is embarrassed by her peculiar tendency to collapse on the floor whenever she feels strong emotion. Since this disorder is caused by REM sleep intrusion during daytime, a neurologist prescribes a medication that reduces and delays REM sleep. Which of the following medications did the neurologist most likely prescribe?

a. Clonazepam
b. Methylphenidate
c. Pimozide
d. Desipramine
e. L-dopa

Questions 477 and 478

477. A mentally retarded male adolescent who has been increasingly aggressive and agitated receives several consecutive IM doses of haloperidol, totaling 30 mg in 24 hours, as a chemical restraint. The next day, he is rigid, confused, and unresponsive. His blood pressure is 150/95 mm Hg, his pulse is 110 beats/minute, and his temperature is 38.9°C (102°F). Both his WBC count and CPK levels are very high. Which of the following is the most likely diagnosis?

a. Acute dystonic reaction
b. Neuroleptic-induced Parkinson disease
c. Malignant hyperthermia
d. Neuroleptic malignant syndrome
e. Catatonia

478. Which of the following medications can be effective in treating the condition in the vignette above?

a. Bromocriptine
b. Carbamazepine
c. Chlorpromazine
d. Lithium
e. Propranolol

479. A 7-year-old boy who wets the bed at least three times a week and has not responded to appropriate behavioral interventions is diagnosed with ADHD. Which of the following medications is indicated to treat both disorders?

a. Bupropion
b. Dextroamphetamine
c. Clonidine
d. Risperidone
e. Imipramine

480. A 47-year-old man comes to a physician for treatment of his impotence. He has had a 20-year history of IDDM, well-controlled, and a 12-year history of alcohol dependence, though he has been sober for 3 years. He is prescribed sildenafil. Which of the following adverse effects is most commonly associated with this drug?

a. Hypoglycemia
b. Ketoacidosis
c. Liver failure
d. Myocardial infarction
e. Arteritic anterior ischemic optic neuropathy (NAION)

481. Which of the following cardiovascular effects can be most problematic secondary to TCA use?

a. Decreased myocardial contractility
b. Slowing of cardiac conduction
c. Increased risk for cardiac ischemia
d. Toxic myocardiopathy
e. Thickening of mitral valve cusps

Questions 482 to 485

For each patient's symptoms, select the most likely diagnosis. Each option can be chosen once, more than once, or not at all.

a. Parkinsonian tremor
b. Akathisia
c. Neuroleptic malignant syndrome
d. Dystonia
e. Anticholinergic syndrome
f. Seizure activity
g. Rabbit syndrome
h. Lithium-induced tremor
i. Akinesia

482. A 35-year-old painter is very frustrated by a fine tremor of her hands that worsens when she works and causes her to smudge her paintings. She was started on a medication several months ago after she had begun to believe that she was the "next Picasso." During that time, she was also hypersexual and bought a car on her husband's credit card.

483. An 18-year-old man is admitted to a locked psychiatric unit after he assaulted his father. He is convinced that his family members have been replaced with malevolent aliens and hears several voices that comment on his actions and call him demeaning names. Two days after initiating treatment, he develops a painful spasm of the neck muscles and his eyes are forced into an upward gaze.

484. A 55-year-old man was diagnosed with a mental illness at the age of 20. At that time, he was noted to have hallucinations of two men commenting on his behavior and delusions that God was going to punish him for not finishing college. Once started on medications, the hallucinations and delusions lessened, though he remained socially isolative and apathetic. After 35 years on the same medication, he has a coarse, pill-rolling tremor that worsens at rest and improves during voluntary movements.

485. A 45-year-old woman with schizoaffective disorder has received neuroleptic medications, antidepressants, and mood stabilizers for at least 20 years. She presents with very rapid chewing movements. Other facial muscles, her trunk, and extremities are not affected, and her tongue does not dart in and out of her mouth when she is asked to protrude it.

Psychopharmacology and Other Somatic Therapies

Answers

430 and 431. The answers are 430-c, 431-e. *(Kaplan and Sadock, p 378.)* The antiretroviral agents have many side effects. They are metabolized by the hepatic cytochrome P450 oxidase system, and can therefore increase the circulating levels of many psychotropic drugs which are metabolized the same way. These include bupropion, meperidine, various benzodiazepines, and SSRIs.

432. The answer is b. *(Kaplan and Sadock, p 257.)* Because of the risk of hypothyroidism that can result from taking Lithium, patients are advised to have a TSH level drawn every 6 months. Also every 6 months, patients should have the signs and symptoms of both hyper- and hypothyroidism reviewed with them, to double check that they are not experiencing any of the symptoms. T3RU and BUN blood tests should be repeated yearly on patients taking Lithium.

433. The answer is c. *(Moore and Jefferson, pp 138-139.)* The SSRIs, including fluoxetine, paroxetine, sertraline, fluvoxamine, and citalopram are well tolerated by the elderly, as are unique agents such as bupropion, venlafaxine, nefazodone, and mirtazapine. The tricyclic drugs include imipramine, desipramine, amitriptyline, and nortriptyline. They are effective in the treatment of depression; several anxiety disorders including panic disorder, generalized anxiety disorder, and separation anxiety; enuresis; and ADHD. Tricyclic antidepressants have different side effect profiles, with each blocking cholinergic, adrenergic, and histaminic receptors to different degrees. For example, there is less anticholinergic activity with desipramine than with imipramine, and nortriptyline is less likely to cause orthostatic hypotension than amitriptyline. However, all tricyclics are at least somewhat anticholinergic and sedating, and thus should not be used as a first-line treatment for major depression in the elderly. Phenelzine and tranylcypromine are both MAO inhibitors, whose major side effect is hypotension—again, not something to be used in the geriatric population, if at all possible.

434. The answer is b. (*Kaplan and Sadock, pp 1111-1112.*) Clomipramine is a tricyclic antidepressant effective in the treatment of obsessive-compulsive disorder in both children and adults. Its efficacy is thought to be related to its effects on inhibition of serotonin reuptake. SSRIs are also effective medications for the treatment of OCD.

435. The answer is d. (*Kaplan and Sadock, pp 1099-1101.*) This young boy suffers from attention deficit hyperactivity disorder (ADHD). The treatment of choice for ADHD is CNS stimulants, primarily detroamphetamine, methylphenidate, and pemoline.

436. The answer is a. (*Kaplan and Sadock, p 259.*) A mild leukopenia (WBC = 3000-3500), with or without clinical symptoms such as lethargy, fever, sore throat, or weakness, should cause the psychiatrist to monitor the patient closely and institute a minimum of twice-weekly CBC tests with differentials included. More serious leucopenia (WBC = 2000-3000) should cause psychiatrists to get daily CBCs and stop the clozapine. It may be reinstituted after the WBCs normalize. With an uncomplicated agranulocytosis (no signs of infection), the patient should be placed in protective isolation, the clozapine should be discontinued, and a bone marrow specimen may need to be gotten to see if progenitor cells are being suppressed. Clozapine must not be restarted in this latter case.

437. The answer is b. (*Jacobson and Jacobson, p 437.*) In cases of mild to moderate lithium toxicity (generally serum levels below 3 meq/L with symptoms of tremor, mild confusion, and gastrointestinal distress), treatment is generally supportive, including IV saline and monitoring of urine output and frequent lithium levels. In more extreme cases, such as this one, the emergency use of dialysis is indicated.

438 and 439. The answers are 438-a, 439-c. (*Kaplan and Sadock, pp 1063-1064.*) Ramelteon mimics melatonin's sleep-inducing properties. It has a high affinity for melatonin MT1 and MT2 receptors in the brain. The half-life of ramelteon is between 1 and 2.5 hours. Ramelteon reduces time to sleep onset, and to a lesser extent, increases the amount of time spent in sleep. The most common side effect is headache. It should not be used in patients with severe hepatic impairment, severe sleep apnea, or severe COPD. There has been no evidence found of rebound insomnia or withdrawal effects from this drug.

440. The answer is c. *(Kaplan and Sadock, p 260.)* Carbamazepine can cause aplastic anemia, agranulocytosis, thrombocytopenia, and leucopenia. It also has a risk of hepatotoxicity. Because of these possible side effects, a CBC, platelet count, reticulocyte count, serum electrolytes, SGOT, SGPT, LDH, and a pregnancy test (in appropriate patients, since carbamazepine raises the risk a baby will be born with spina bifida) should all be drawn before treatment with carbamazepine is instituted. SGOT, SGPT, and LDP should be drawn every month for the first 2 months, and thereafter, every 3 months.

441. The answer is c. *(Kaplan and Sadock, pp 406, 449, 458.)* This patient's respiration is very depressed, and it is likely that the benzodiazepines are playing a role. Flumazenil can be used in the emergency room setting to counteract the effects of benzodiazepine overdose. LAAM is an opioid agonist that suppresses opioid withdrawal. It is no longer used, because patients developed prolonged QT intervals associated with potentially fatal arrhythmias. Disulfiram is used as an aversive treatment to maintain sobriety in those with alcohol dependence, and acamprosate is also used to improve treatment outcomes in those with alcoholism, though the exact treatment mechanism is not known.

442. The answer is b. *(Kaplan and Sadock, p 626.)* It is unlikely that this patient will respond to the use of buspirone, because she has previously been using benzodiazepines. The lack of response may be caused by the absence of some of the nonanxiolytic effects of benzodiazepines as opposed to buspirone, that is, because the patient has become used to the muscle relaxant and general sense of well-being effects of the benzodiazepines, she may well fail to see the treatment effects of buspirone, which tend to be more effective in reducing the cognitive symptoms of GAD over the somatic symptoms anyway.

443 and 444. The answers are 443-b, 444-d. *(Kaplan and Sadock, pp 100-103.)* Dopamine receptor blockade causes hyperprolactinemia, which in turn can cause breast enlargement, galactorrhea (abnormal discharge of milk from the breast), and suppression of testosterone production in men. The typical neuroleptics (eg, haloperidol and chlorpromazine) are particularly prone to causing these side effects.

445. The answer is e. (*Kaplan and Sadock, p 744.*) Sertraline would be the best choice for this woman, who is determined not to gain back the 50 lb she has lost. Amitriptyline is associated with a great tendency to gain weight, while doxepin, nortriptyline, and phenelzine all have an intermediate tendency to increase appetite and body weight.

446. The answer is b. (*Kaplan and Sadock, pp 850-851.*) St. John's wort is used as an antidepressant, a sedative, and an anxiolytic. Ginseng is used as a stimulant, for fatigue, the elevation of mood, and to improve the functioning of the immune system.

447. The answer is a. (*Kaplan and Sadock, p 867.*) The FDA rates drugs for their safety of use during pregnancy. Category A drugs have shown no fetal risks in controlled studies and consist of drugs such as iron. Category B drugs have shown no fetal risk in animal studies, but there have been no controlled human studies (or have shown fetal risk in animals, but no risk in well-controlled human studies). Drugs in this category include Tylenol. Category C drugs have shown adverse fetal effects in animals, with no human data available. Drugs in this category include aspirin, haloperidol, and chlorpromazine. Category D drugs have shown human fetal risk, but may be used in life-threatening situations. These drugs include lithium, tetracycline, and ethanol. Category X drugs, of which valproic acid and thalidomide are examples, have shown proven fetal risk and should not be used in any circumstances by pregnant women.

448. The answer is b. (*Kaplan and Sadock, p 260.*) Aplastic anemia is a rare, idiosyncratic, non-dose-related side effect of carbamazepine. Stevens-Johnson syndrome is a potentially life-threatening exfoliative dermatitis, also rarely associated with carbamazepine treatment that usually develops shortly after starting the drug. Neuroleptic malignant syndrome, serotonin syndrome, and malignant hyperthermia are not associated with this medication.

449. The answer is b. (*Kaplan and Sadock, p 916.*) This patient is suffering from neuroleptic malignant syndrome. This disorder presents with hyperthermia, muscle rigidity, autonomic instability, and has a 10% to 30% fatality rate. Creatine phosphokinase can be tremendously elevated because of the extreme muscle rigidity that can be seen, and should be carefully monitored. The offending antipsychotic should be discontinued, the patient should be hydrated and cooled, and dantrolene (IV) and/or bromocriptine (orally) may be given.

450. The answer is b. (*Kaplan and Sadock, p 914.*) This patient is suffering from a moderately severe acute dystonia, which can be very uncomfortable. The patient should be given benztropine or diphenhydramine IM in an emergency room setting, to decrease the amount of time spent suffering with the dystonia. If possible longer term, the offending antipsychotic should be decreased, and benztropine or diphenhydramine can be prescribed po to prevent a recurrence.

451. The answer is a. (*Jacobson and Jacobson, p 178.*) Phenothiazines, tricyclic anti-depressants, and antiparkinsonian agents (such as benztropine mesylate) all have anticholinergic properties. The action of these drugs becomes additive when they are administered in combination. It is not uncommon for persons receiving such a combination to show evidence of a mild organic brain syndrome, including difficulty in concentrating; impaired short-term memory; disorientation, which often is more noticeable at night; and dry skin caused by inhibition of sweating.

452. The answer is e. (*Kaplan and Sadock, p 918.*) Discontinuation of the antipsychotic medication or a dosage decrease are the initial interventions recommended when tardive dyskinesia is first diagnosed. If discontinuation is not possible and dosage decrease is not effective, clozapine has been proven effective in ameliorating and suppressing the symptoms of tardive dyskinesia.

453. The answer is c. (*Kaplan and Sadock, p 983.*) In 2007, the FDA reported the presence of an idiosyncratic drug response to certain sedative-hypnotics in a small percentage of patients, causing a dissociative-like state. During these states, patient had episodes of sleepwalking, binge-eating, aggressive outbursts, and night driving, all during which the patient was completely unaware of the behavior. Zolpidem and Zaleplon are now both required to have warning labels to this effect.

454. The answer is e. (*Kaplan and Sadock, p 993.*) This patient is suffering from akathisia, which is a subjective feeling of restlessness, coupled with the need to move. Patients may rock, pace, sit, and stand back and forth, or generally appear jittery. Once it has been recognized, the offending antipsychotic should be reduced as much as possible. The most efficacious drugs are β-adrenergic receptor antagonists like propranolol, though benzodiazepines and anticholinergics may also be somewhat effective.

455. The answer is e. (*Kaplan and Sadock, pp 1117-1124.*) This man is clearly suffering from a very severe major depression, and has already had one serious suicide attempt. Refusing to eat or drink means that he needs an effective treatment for his depression that will work very quickly. In this case ECT should be the treatment of choice.

456. The answer is c. (*Kaplan and Sadock, p 1014.*) Methohexital is commonly used for ECT. It has lower cardiac risks than other barbiturates. Used IV, it produces rapid unconsciousness and patients reawaken quickly thereafter, since the duration of action is only 5 to 7 minutes.

457. The answer is e. (*Kaplan and Sadock, pp 1106-1113.*) Urinary retention, blurred vision, constipation, and dry mouth are common anticholinergic side effects associated with tricyclic antidepressants. Among these medications, amitriptyline is the most anticholinergic. Venlafaxine, bupropion, trazodone, and nefazodone do not have significant anticholinergic effects.

458. The answer is b. (*Kaplan and Sadock, p 1024.*) Bupropion may be helpful to patients with hypoactive sexual desire disorder, and is also used to help patients stop smoking, when combined with a structured behavioral support system. This patient may benefit from this single drug to treat both of her problems.

459. The answer is b. (*Kaplan and Sadock, pp 1098-1103.*) Ritalin is well known to cause insomnia, and thus should not be given after noon. Other side effects may include a reduced appetite, headache, gastrointestinal upset, and the emergence of tics.

460 and 461. The answers are 460-b, 461-e. (*Kaplan and Sadock, p 406.*) Disulfiram inhibits acetaldehyde dehydrogenase, one of the main enzymes in the metabolism of ethyl alcohol. Ingestion of alcohol, even in small quantities, causes accumulation of toxic acetaldehyde and a variety of unpleasant symptoms, including facial flushing, tachycardia, vomiting, and nausea. Many over-the-counter cough and cold medications contain as much as 40% alcohol and can precipitate such a reaction. The intensity of the disulfiram-alcohol interaction varies with each patient and with the quantity of alcohol consumed. Extreme cases are characterized by respiratory depression, seizures, cardiovascular collapse, and even death. For this reason, the use of disulfiram is recommended only with highly motivated patients who will agree to carefully avoid any food or medication containing alcohol.

462. The answer is c. (*Kaplan and Sadock, pp 759-760.*) There is no cure for narcolepsy, but stimulants such as methylphenidate, pemoline, and amphetamine can ameliorate daytime sleepiness. Medications that reduce REM sleep, such as TCAs and SSRIs, are used if cataplexy is also present. Modafinil has recently been approved by the FDA to reduce the number of sleep attacks and to improve psychomotor performance in narcolepsy.

463. The answer is d. (*Kaplan and Sadock, pp 328-329.*) Clozapine is the preferred treatment for psychotic symptoms in patients with Parkinson disease. Because of its relative sparing of the nigrostriatal dopaminergic system and its anti-cholinergic effects, clozapine does not worsen and may in fact ameliorate parkinsonian symptoms. Typical antipsychotic medications, on the contrary, tend to aggravate the extrapyramidal symptoms of patients with Parkinson disease.

464. The answer is b. (*Kaplan and Sadock, p 1032.*) Of the medicines listed in the options to this question, only erythromycin can increase the plasma concentration of carbamazepine. Theophylline and cisplatin can decrease carbamazepine levels. Hormonal contraceptives and warfarin can have their levels decreased by the presence of carbamazepine.

465. The answer is c. (*Kaplan and Sadock, pp 1056-1063.*) Since the half-life of lithium is about 20 hours, equilibrium is reached after 5 to 7 days of regular intake. (Steady state is reached after approximately five half-lives of the drug being administered.)

466. The answer is b. (*Kaplan and Sadock, pp 1000-1003.*) Propranolol and other beta-blockers can be used to treat akathisia, which this patient seems to demonstrate. Since beta-receptor blockade causes bronchospasm, these medications are contraindicated in patients with asthma. If this patient had asthma, a better treatment for her akathisia might be a benzodiazepine (although this drug might be problematic for a patient with a substance abuse history).

467. The answer is d. (*Kaplan and Sadock, pp 1103-1105.*) The connection between thyroid function and mood disorders has been known for more than a century, since nineteenth-century physicians noticed that hypothyroidism was accompanied by depression. All the hormones of the hypothalamic-pituitary-thyroid axis have been used in the treatment of depression, alone or in combination with other agents, although the most commonly used are liothyronine and levothyroxine.

468. The answer is e. (*Kaplan and Sadock, p 1093.*) The patient should have the clozapine temporarily discontinued and phenobarbital begun. The occurrence of seizures during clozapine treatment is dose related and increases considerably with dosages greater than 400 mg/day. Phenobarbital is considered the safest and the best-tolerated anticonvulsant for patients taking clozapine who experience seizures. It should be started after clozapine is stopped; then the clozapine can be restarted at 50% of its previous dosage and gradually raised. Carbamazepine should be avoided because the bone marrow suppression risk with this medication can increase the risk for agranulocytosis with clozapine.

469. The answer is a. (*Kaplan and Sadock, p 557.*) Patients with seasonal depression and bipolar depression with a seasonal component can benefit from exposure to bright light, in the range of 1500 to 10,000 lux or more for 1 to 2 hours every day before dawn. Phototherapy is effective alone in mild cases and as an adjunct to medication treatment in more severe cases.

470. The answer is a. (*Kaplan and Sadock, p 621.*) Practically every class of medication has been used to treat posttraumatic stress disorder, including every family of antidepressant, mood stabilizers, anxiolytics, and inhibitors of adrenergic activity, such as clonidine and propranolol. Clonidine and beta-blockers can be particularly useful, alone or in combination with other medications, to treat symptoms of hyperarousal. These drugs block the adrenergic symptoms of hyperarousal, which in turn may allow patients with PTSD to better control feelings of anger, rage, or panic.

471. The answer is d. (*Kaplan and Sadock, p 1357.*) High-potency neuroleptics, such as haloperidol and fluphenazine, being low in anticholinergic side effects and less likely to cause postural hypotension, are preferred to low-potency medications such as chlorpromazine in elderly patients with cardiovascular problems and prostatic hypertrophy. Clozapine is not recommended because of its powerful anticholinergic effects, its tendency to cause hypotension, and the risk for agranulocytosis. Thioridazine is the least appropriate medication in this case because, aside from sharing the side effects profile of the other low-potency neuroleptics, it can cause fatal arrhythmias by prolonging the QT interval. Finally, olanzapine is not appropriate for this patient because it causes significant postural hypotension.

472. The answer is c. (*Kaplan and Sadock, p 1089.*) Abrupt discontinuation of an SSRI causes a variety of symptoms that can be quite distressing for the patient. The most common physical symptoms are dizziness, nausea, vomiting, lethargy, flu-like symptoms (chills and aches), and sensory and sleep disturbances. Commonly reported psychological symptoms are irritability, anxiety, and crying spells. Symptoms usually emerge 1 to 3 days after the last dose. Paroxetine and sertraline, because of their shorter half-life, are the SSRIs most likely to cause a discontinuation syndrome and should be tapered off over several weeks. Owing to its long half-life and its active metabolites, fluoxetine can be stopped abruptly without problems.

473. The answer is a. (*Kaplan and Sadock, p 1018.*) Benzodiazepines bind to GABA receptors, which represent the main cortical and thalamic inhibitory system and potentiate the response of these receptors to GABA. Benzodiazepines do not have any direct effect on the GABA receptors unless GABA is present.

474 and 475. The answers are 474-a, 475-a. (*Kaplan and Sadock, pp 1067-1068.*) Over-the-counter medications containing sympathomimetic agents such as pseudoephedrine can cause severe hypertensive crises in patients on MAOIs because of the inhibition of their main metabolic pathway. Tyramine, a powerful hypertensive agent, is contained in many foods and is usually metabolized by monoamine oxidase. Foods to be avoided by patients on MAOIs include tyramine-rich foods such as aged cheese, salami, pepperoni, sausage, overripe fruit, liquors, red wine, pickled fish, sauerkraut, and brewer's yeast. Chocolate, coffee, tea, beer, and white wine can be consumed in small quantities. Nonaged cheeses like cream cheese or cottage cheese may be consumed without difficulty.

476. The answer is d. (*Kaplan and Sadock, pp 759-760.*) Many antidepressants, including SSRIs, TCAs, and MAOIs, suppress REM sleep and can be useful in the treatment of cataplexy. The other medications listed do not affect sleep cycles.

477 and 478. The answers are 477-d, 478-a. (*Moore and Jefferson, pp 265-266.*) Neuroleptic malignant syndrome (NMS) is a relatively rare but potentially fatal complication of neuroleptic treatment. Its main features are hyperthermia, severe muscular rigidity, autonomic instability, and changes in mental status. Associated findings are increased CPK, increased liver transaminase activity, leukocytes, and myoglobinuria. The mortality rate can be as high as 30% and can be higher when the syndrome is precipitated by depot forms. Neuroleptic malignant syndrome is more common in young males when high-potency neuroleptics are used in high doses and when dosage is escalated rapidly. The first step in management of NMS is discontinuation of all antipsychotic medications. Supportive treatments include treatment of extrapyramidal symptoms with antiparkinson medications, correcting fluid imbalances, treating fever, and managing hypertension or hypotension. Dopaminergic agents such as dantrolene, bromocriptine, and amantidine are used in the treatment of more severe cases.

479. The answer is e. (*Moore and Jefferson, pp 323-326.*) Imipramine is effective in the treatment of nocturnal enuresis, through a still unknown mechanism. Its beneficial effects in this disorder may be related to its anticholinergic properties or an effect on the sleep process. Imipramine is also used with good results in the treatment of children and adults with ADHD, although it is not as effective as the stimulants. Imipramine can be helpful for patients with comorbid anxiety or tics, patients who do not tolerate stimulants, or patients who have a history of substance abuse.

480. The answer is d. (*Kaplan and Sadock, pp 1079-1080.*) The most important adverse side effect associated with sildenafil is myocardial infarction. While the drugs themselves do not posed an increased risk of death in this manner, the increased oxygen demand and stress placed on the heart by sexual activity, in a heart that is already affected by an underlying condition such as atherosclerotic disease may precipitate a heart attack.

Non-arteritic anterior ischemic optic neuropathy (NAION) is a very rare but serious condition which may occur in men taking sildenafil. It causes restriction of blood flow to the optic nerve and can result in permanent blindness.

481. The answer is b. *(Kaplan and Sadock, p 1110.)* Tricyclic antidepressants have a quinidine-like antiarrhythmic effect and slow cardiac conduction. Although at therapeutic dosages they may have a beneficial effect on ventricular excitability, in patients with preexisting prolonged QRS or in any person at toxic dosages, TCAs can cause a fatal heart block. TCAs do not affect cardiac contractility or cardiac output, nor do they cause cardiomyopathy or valvular deformities.

482 to 485. The answers are 482-h, 483-d, 484-a, 485-g. *(Kaplan and Sadock, pp 976-1112.)* Lithium causes a benign, high-frequency, fine tremor that worsens during activities requiring fine motor control. Dose reduction, elimination of caffeine, slow-release lithium preparations, and beta-blockers are the main therapeutic interventions. A severe tremor at any time during lithium treatment may be a sign of toxicity. Neuroleptic-induced dystonia is characterized by intermittent or sustained muscle spasms, usually involving the head and neck. Common symptoms include torticollis (neck spasms), tongue spasms that interfere with speech, and oculogyric crises (eyes forced in an upward gaze). Opisthotonus can also occur, but is less frequent. Dystonic reactions are more common in young males at the beginning of the treatment and when high-potency neuroleptics are used. Anticholinergic medications such as benztropine and diphenhydramine, administered intramuscularly, are the treatments of choice. Coarse, pill-rolling, nonintentional tremor that improves with intentional movement and worsens at rest is characteristic of Parkinson disease and neuroleptic-induced parkinsonianism. Cogwheel rigidity, a stiff gait with short steps, and expressionless face and speech are other common parkinsonian symptoms. Rabbit syndrome is an uncommon extrapyramidal neuroleptic-induced syndrome often confused with tardive dyskinesia. In this syndrome, the chewing movements are much more rapid and regular than the orofacial choreoathetoid movements typical of tardive dyskinesia. Furthermore, the tongue and other parts of the body are not involved. While uncommon, it is distressing to patients, and it may respond to anticholinergic agents.

Law and Ethics in Psychiatry

Questions

486. In order to successfully sue for medical malpractice, a plaintiff must prove four elements. Three of these elements are negligent performance of patient care, harm to the patient as a direct result of the physician's actions, and damage or harm to the patient. Which of the following is the fourth element?

a. The patient was not informed of the actions the physician was taking.
b. The patient was not in agreement with the treatment plan.
c. Notes were not kept in an orderly and complete fashion.
d. There was a duty on the part of the physician to treat the patient.
e. There was intent to harm the patient.

487. A 56-year-old woman in the last stages of amyotrophic lateral sclerosis asks for her life support to be stopped and to be allowed to die. Her family members disagree with her decision and go to court to keep the patient alive. A psychiatric evaluation finds the patient mentally sound and fully able to understand the consequences of her decision. Which of the following actions should be taken next?

a. The family's desires overrule the patient's wishes, so the patient's life support should be continued.
b. Terminating one's life is illegal, so the patient's life support should be continued.
c. A guardian must be appointed to make decisions on behalf of the patient so that a neutral third party can decide this issue.
d. Since the patient's life expectancy is more than 2 weeks, she cannot be allowed to die and her life support should be continued.
e. The patient is competent, and as such she has the right to refuse unwanted medical treatment—her life support should be withdrawn.

Questions 488 and 489

488. An emaciated 26-year-old man is brought to the emergency room by the local police late one night in the dead of winter. The police tell the psychiatrist on call that the man was preaching loudly at a nearby busy intersection, sometimes walking into traffic to approach drivers while dressed only in a thin robe despite the freezing temperatures. On interview, the psychiatrist notes that the man displays delusions of special connections to God and discounts any concern for his physical safety, as he will leave his fate to God. The patient refuses voluntary admission, stating that he must get back to his divine mission. On what grounds would the emergency room psychiatrist be most justified in hospitalizing the patient involuntarily?

a. The patient is so disorganized as to be unable to attend to his basic physical needs.
b. The patient is suffering from acute psychosis.
c. The patient is at risk for causing harm to other people.
d. The patient's psychiatric disorder is likely to worsen in the future without treatment.
e. The patient's behavior could be interpreted as actively suicidal.

489. The patient in the vignette above is admitted to the hospital involuntarily. On the inpatient unit, he is noted to be mild-mannered and soft-spoken. He refuses all forms of treatment, stating that God is his only healer. While the patient is not particularly disruptive and not aggressive in any way, staff are nevertheless concerned about his refusal of treatment. In fact, he is noted to be trying very persistently to "convert" the other patients and staff on the unit, sometimes to their marked irritation. A decision is made by the staff to medicate the patient against his will. Subsequently, members of the patient's family bring suit against the clinical team working with the patient. On what grounds would the lawsuit initiated by the family most likely be brought?

a. The involuntary treatment violated the family's constitutional rights.
b. The treatment violated the family's religious beliefs.
c. The patient had a right to refuse treatment because he was not in any immediate danger.
d. The treatment could have caused side effects.
e. The patient did not have a history of aggressive behavior.

490. A 46-year-old man is on a ventilator and has been irreversibly and severely brain damaged as a result of a motorcycle accident. Prior to the crash, he had told his wife during conversations about this kind of incapacity that he would not wish to have the life support withdrawn because he said he had "seen stories of medical miracles occurring where people awoke from these states." He had not, however, signed a living will. The patient's parents are requesting that the life support be withdrawn because they cannot bear to see their son existing in this manner. Which of the following actions should be taken (and why), given these circumstances?

a. The life support should be withdrawn because the parents wish it and no living will has been signed by the patient.
b. The life support should be withdrawn because there is no hope of the patient's recovery.
c. The life support should be continued because the patient's wishes are clearly known, even though there is no living will.
d. The life support should be continued because in the absence of a living will, a hospital will get sued if it is withdrawn.
e. The case should be heard in front of a court so that the decision can be made by a neutral third party.

491. A 4-year-old boy is brought to the emergency room by his mother secondary to a fracture of his left femur. The mother states that the boy fell down the stairs at home, and that he has "always been clumsy." X-rays of the boy's leg confirm the fracture, and physical examination reveals bruises of various ages on the boy's chest and abdomen. Which of the following should the physician do first?

a. Arrange for a comprehensive psychiatric evaluation of the child.
b. Ensure the child's safety.
c. Report the case to the appropriate child-family social service department.
d. Order a complete skeletal survey (x-rays) of the child.
e. Request social work intervention.

492. The landmark decision in Tarasoff I held that a therapist has an obligation to do which of the following?

a. Protect the confidentiality of information obtained during therapy.
b. Notify the police when a patient is involved in illegal activities.
c. Report a minor's sexual activity to the patient's parents.
d. Warn the potential victim of a potentially violent patient.
e. Seek informed consent from patients who are given neuroleptic medications.

493. Which of the following is the most common cause of malpractice claims in psychiatric practice?

a. Improper treatment resulting in physical injury
b. Homicide
c. Sexual involvement between physician and patient
d. Failure to treat psychosis
e. Improper certification in hospitalization

494. A 63-year-old physician comes to a psychiatrist because he "just can't handle it anymore." The physician states he had to tell a patient that she is dying, and it "tore him apart." He is concerned that he will be unable to care for this patient well because his own feelings keep getting in the way. Which of the following best describes a risk factor for physicians to develop such aversive reactions to the care of dying patients?

a. The physician feels professionally secure.
b. The physician has a healthy extended family.
c. The physician can tolerate high levels of ambiguity.
d. The physician identifies the patient with someone in his own life.
e. The physician has resolved grief issues.

495. Which of the following statements refers to the principle of beneficence?

a. Prevent harm and promote well-being
b. Do no harm
c. Treat indigent patients without monetary compensation
d. Provide universal health care
e. Build the patient-doctor relationship on trust

496. In Tarasoff II, the second decision by the California Supreme Court on the case, the original Tarasoff ruling was revised by the addition of which of the following?

a. Requiring the warning of only identifiable potential victims
b. Imposing legal liability on police
c. Requiring hospitalization of patients deemed dangerous
d. Instituting a duty to protect potential victims, not just warn them
e. Requiring use of neuroleptic medication to treat potentially dangerous patients

497. A 57-year-old man is seeing a psychiatrist for the treatment of his major depression. During the course of his treatment, the man describes in great detail the fact that he has molested several children. Some of these molestations occurred decades previously, but one, according to the patient, is ongoing, involving a 10-year-old boy who lives in an apartment next door to the patient. Which of the following actions should the psychiatrist take next?

a. The psychiatrist should take no action outside the therapeutic setting but, rather, try to explore the unconscious determinants of this patient's behavior.
b. The psychiatrist should take no action outside the therapeutic setting because the patient is protected by confidentiality laws.
c. The psychiatrist should admit the patient to a psychiatric hospital and call the boy's parents to alert them to the danger.
d. The psychiatrist should call the police and have them apprehend the patient at the next treatment session.
e. The psychiatrist should immediately report the patient's behavior to the appropriate state agency.

498. A 24-year-old woman sues her psychiatrist for abandonment because he retired from practice. She states that her mental condition has deteriorated significantly since he left because he had provided her care for over 5 years and knew her "better than anyone." She states that the psychiatrist gave her 6 months' notice of his retirement and gave her the names of four psychiatrists whom he had determined had treatment openings for new patients. She states that she had seen one of the psychiatrists on the list 1 month after her original psychiatrist retired, but that this new psychiatrist did not know her very well. Which of the following is the most likely outcome of this lawsuit?

a. The psychiatrist will be found guilty of dereliction of duty.
b. The psychiatrist will be found guilty of abandonment because he did not give notice of his retirement early enough.
c. The psychiatrist will be found not guilty of abandonment but will be censored for unethical treatment of his patient.
d. The psychiatrist will be found not guilty of abandonment, since he provided his patient with reasonable notice and a reasonable effort to find her a new therapist.
e. The psychiatrist will be found guilty of abandonment because he did not make sure that his patient had actually seen another psychiatrist before his retirement.

499. A 78-year-old man chooses his wife to be his surrogate for decision making because he has been diagnosed with Alzheimer disease and knows that he will not be capable of making such decisions in the future. Two years later, the disease is fairly advanced, and the patient is hallucinating at night, which often disrupts his ability to sleep. The patient's physician recommends a low dose of an antipsychotic medication for the patient. How should the patient's wife make the decision whether or not to have the medication administered?

a. The wife should use her own best judgment based on what she would want done for herself in the same situation.
b. The wife should use substituted judgment, which requires her to decide what to do, based on what the patient would have wished if he were capable of making the decision.
c. The wife should use the best-interests approach, which means that she should make the decision based on what could reasonably be assumed to be in the patient's best interest.
d. The wife should follow the physician's recommendation, whatever it is, because the physician can be assumed to have the patient's best interests at heart.
e. The wife should consult with another physician about the use of a new medication before she makes any decisions.

500. In which of the following situations, if confidentiality were broken, could an individual patient sue and likely win the case?

a. A trainee discussing his patient's psychotherapy with a supervisor.
b. A communicable disease is reported to an authorized public health authority.
c. In an emergency situation, to prevent an imminent threat to the safety of a person.
d. To report the victim of abuse or neglect.
e. Reporting of a patient's psychotherapy in detail for a journal article.

Law and Ethics in Psychiatry

Answers

486. The answer is d. *(Kaplan and Sadock, p 1371.)* In a malpractice lawsuit, the plaintiff must show by a preponderance of evidence that the four elements of malpractice are present. These are the so-called four Ds of malpractice: (1) a duty existed toward the patient on the part of the psychiatrist, (2) a deviation from the standard of practice occurred, (3) this deviation bore a direct causal relationship to the untoward outcome, and (4) damages occurred as a result.

487. The answer is e. *(Kaplan and Sadock, pp 1375-1376.)* Nancy Cruzan had been in a vegetative state, kept alive by feeding tubes, for over 4 years. Because her prognosis was hopeless, her parents went to court to have the feeding stopped so that she could die. The case ultimately found its way to the Supreme Court, which ruled that competent persons have a constitutional right to refuse unwanted medical treatment (Cruzan v. Director). The court left it to the states to decide how to handle the situation of the incompetent patient, and in many states that has limited the rights of families to make decisions unless there is an advance directive such as a living will or a durable power of attorney. In this case, the patient is competent, so the life support should be withdrawn as she requests.

488. The answer is a. *(Kaplan and Sadock, pp 1374-1375.)* The emergency room psychiatrist was justified in hospitalizing the patient involuntarily because the patient appeared to be mentally ill and unable to care for his own basic needs. In this case, being properly clothed to avoid the potential harmful effects of exposure to cold would be considered a basic need. The essential criteria that must be met in order for an involuntary hospitalization to be justified are as follows: (1) there must be evidence of the presence of mental illness, (2) the patient must be at risk for causing imminent harm to him- or herself or to others, and (3) the patient must be unable to provide for his or her basic needs. In the absence of strong evidence for imminent danger or risk of harm to self or others, patients maintain the right to refuse treatment, even when they have been hospitalized involuntarily.

489. The answer is c. *(Kaplan and Sadock, pp 1375-1376.)* Since the patient was residing in a hospital unit at the time the unwanted treatments were administered, he was at no immediate risk of the sort that originally led to his admission. Nor was there any evidence that he was acting in ways that placed himself or others in immediate danger or at risk of harm. The family's beliefs and rights are not relevant in this context.

490. The answer is c. *(Kaplan and Sadock, pp 1375-1376.)* This patient has made his wishes clearly known; therefore, even in the absence of a living will, those wishes should be followed. In the case where the wishes have not been clearly communicated, hospitals may carry out their interest in "the protection and preservation of human life" by denying requests from others (even family members) for discontinuing life support. In 1990, the Supreme Court upheld the right of a competent person to have a "constitutionally protected liberty interest in refusing unwanted medical treatment." The Supreme Court applied this principle to all patients who have made their wishes clearly known, whether or not they ever become conscious.

491. The answer is b. *(Kaplan and Sadock, p 880.)* The first and foremost action that should be taken in this situation is to make sure that the child is safe. This may mean that the child must be removed from the family. All the other options as answers to this question may at some time be advisable, but not until the safety of the child is at first taken care of.

492. The answer is d. *(Kaplan and Sadock, pp 1373-1374.)* The Tarasoff decision was a landmark case in determining that psychotherapists have an obligation to warn third parties who are in danger. In this instance, the therapist had an obligation to warn the potential victim of a student who had threatened to kill the girl who had rejected him. The patient ultimately killed the girl, thus prompting the litigation.

493. The answer is a. *(Kaplan and Sadock, pp 1371-1372.)* Improper treatment is the most common reason for malpractice claims in psychiatry, accounting for 33% of all claims. This is followed by attempted or completed suicide, which account for 20% of all claims.

494. The answer is d. *(Kaplan and Sadock, pp 1359-1360.)* Physicians often find themselves in the difficult position of caring for a dying patient. Risk factors for the development of aversive reactions to the care of dying patients include: the physician identifies with the patient or identifies the patient with someone important in his own life; the physician is currently dealing with a sick family member or is recently bereaved; the physician feels professionally insecure; is fearful of death and disability; cannot tolerate high levels of uncertainty or ambiguity; or has his own psychiatric diagnosis such as a major depression or substance abuse. The physician may also be unconsciously reflecting feelings felt by the patient or family.

495. The answer is a. (*Kaplan and Sadock, p 1383.*) The principle of beneficence refers to preventing or removing harm and promoting well-being. This principle, along with that of nonmaleficence (doing no harm), has been, until recently, the primary driving force behind medical and psychiatric practice throughout history. Now economic considerations figure much more prominently than ever before in clinical decision-making. The fiduciary principle states that the doctor-patient relationship is built on a sense of honor and trust that the doctor will act competently and responsibly in partnership with the patient and with the patient's consent. This trust is earned and maintained by continuous attention to the patient's needs, a concept known as responsibility.

496. The answer is d. (*Kaplan and Sadock, p 1374.*) Tarasoff I held that psychotherapists and the police have a duty to warn third parties who are in danger. Tarasoff II stated that once a therapist has reasonably determined that a patient poses a serious danger of violence to others, the therapist "bears a duty to exercise reasonable care to protect the foreseeable victim of that danger." This is an expansion of the more narrow duty to warn; it also exempted the police from liability. There is no explicit requirement for specific treatment, such as medications or hospitalization, though these might well be employed by the psychiatrist in the management of potentially violent persons.

497. The answer is e. (*Kaplan and Sadock, p 1373.*) All states legally require that psychiatrists, upon becoming aware of a child who is the victim of sexual or physical abuse, report it to the appropriate state agency. In this case, some of the abuses occurred decades ago, and as such the victims are now probably adults. These cases would not require reporting to authorities. However, the active molestation of the 10-year-old boy requires reporting, since the harm to vulnerable children is considered to outweigh the rights of confidentiality in a psychiatric setting.

498. The answer is d. (*Kaplan and Sadock, p 1390.*) The psychiatrist in this case has done what is ethically proper in preparation for his retirement. He has notified his patient of the retirement with what can be considered sufficient notice, and he has made reasonable efforts to make sure the patient has follow-up care. Many patients in this scenario will undoubtedly feel abandoned, as they might in cases where the psychiatrist moves or goes on an extended leave of absence, but it is unlikely that the lawsuit based on abandonment in this case would hold up in court.

499. The answer is b. (*Kaplan and Sadock, pp 1371-1381.*) Current autonomy-based legal approaches require surrogate decision makers to make decisions based on the principle of substituted judgment, which means that the decision maker should try to make the decision based on what the patient would do if he or she could make decisions on his or her own. This, of course, requires surrogates to have a very good grasp of the attitudes and wishes of those for whom they are making decisions. In the absence of any idea of what the patient might want, the surrogate should use the best-interests approach, which says that the surrogate should make the decision based on what could reasonably be expected to be in the best interest of the patient in the situation at hand.

500. The answer is e. (*Ebert et al, p 711.*) Patients have a right to privacy of their health-related information, and psychiatric patients have the right to privacy with regards to information they may share in therapy. There are many exceptions to this rule, however. Exceptions may include: during emergency circumstances in which the physician is attempting to prevent a serious and imminent threat to the health of a person or the public; after a general consent is given by the patient, information can be exchanged between health care providers to help facilitate the patient's treatment; trainees discussing their patients' psychotherapy sessions with their supervisors; reporting disease and injuries to authorized public authorities; reporting victims of abuse, neglect, or domestic violence as required by law; and reporting adverse effects to the Food and Drug Administration. While clinicians may share information about their patients with other clinicians to facilitate patient care, it is best to realize that such sharing should be done in an appropriate venue, such as in an office, rather than in the hallway or cafeteria. Sharing a patient's case history through a case report for a journal, but leaving the patient's identifying information intact, would be grounds for a lawsuit.

Bibliography

Ebert MH, Loosen PT, Nurcombe B, et al, eds. *Current Diagnosis and Treatment in Psychiatry*. 2nd ed. New York: McGraw-Hill; 2008.

Jacobson JL, Jacobson AM. *Psychiatric Secrets*. 2nd ed. Philadelphia, PA: Hanley and Belfus; 2001.

Kaplan HI, Sadock BJ. *Synopsis of Psychiatry: Behavioral Sciences/Clinical Psychiatry*. 10th ed. Philadelphia, PA: Lippincott, Williams & Wilkins; 2007.

Moore DP, Jefferson JW. *Handbook of Medical Psychiatry*. 2nd ed. Philadelphia, PA: Mosby; 2004.

Index